Edited by **Barbara Zipser**

Simon of Genoa's
Medical Lexicon

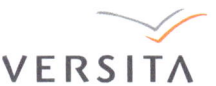

**Versita Discipline:
History, Archaeology**

Managing Editor:
Katarzyna Ślusarska

Language Editor:
Abby Hahn

Published by Versita, Versita Ltd, 78 York Street, London W1H 1DP, Great Britain.

ISBN (hardcover): 978-83-7656-022-9

ISBN (paperback): 978-83-7656-021-2

ISBN (for electronic copy): 978-83-7656-023-6

Managing Editor: Katarzyna Ślusarska

Language Editor: Abby Hahn

Cover illustration: © Bibliothèque Nationale de France, *Par. lat.* 6958, f. 164v.

www.versita.com

Contents

Acknowledgements

The present volume contains the proceedings of the eponymous conference held in central London on the 17th of March 2012. The conference formed part of the *Simon Online* project, a collaborative online edition of Simon of Genoa's *Clavis sanationis*.

The conference, and the resulting publication would not have been possible without the generous support of the Wellcome Trust (Symposia Grant 098262) and the History Department of Royal Holloway University of London. While I organized the conference and edited the book, I was funded by a Wellcome Trust University Award (048921).

I would like to thank Versita for accepting the book for publication, and Katarzyna Ślusarska for seeing it through production. I am also grateful to the Bibliothèque Nationale Paris and the Staatsbibliothek zu Berlin, Preussischer Kulturbesitz who granted permission to publish photographs of their holdings open access. Last but not least I extend my thanks to the authors, the audience at the conference and all those who have contributed to *Simon Online*.

Barbara Zipser, RHUL

Vivian Nutton

Simon of Genoa and Medieval Medicine

The history of medieval medicine has long been tied up with the discovery and editing of texts.

As with medieval history in general, scholars like De Renzi and Daremberg in the mid nineteenth century found it necessary to delve into archives and manuscript collections to supplement what was meagrely available in the form of printed books. The creation of a documentary basis for medicine was one of the central tasks of these pioneers, and was further established from the 1880s onwards by Karl Sudhoff, the dominant figure in the history of medicine for half a century. The pages of *Sudhoffs Archiv* and the *Mitteilungen zur Geschichte der Medizin,* to say nothing of the *Abhandlungen* of his Leipzig Institute, are filled with editions and texts of all kinds, both large and small. Pupils and admirers around Europe followed his example. Even Henry Ernest Sigerist, his Leipzig successor who is now famous for his work on the social aspects of the history of medicine, began his academic career as an editor and cataloguer of medieval texts.

Sudhoff himself concentrated on two sorts of text: tracts and documents relating to the Black Death and other epidemics, and the archival evidence for the development of university medicine. His example laid the foundation for all subsequent studies of medieval ideas on epidemics, as well as of the institutional development of universities across Europe. He was less concerned with the actual university lectures that were delivered (a gap that has only partially been filled since his death), particularly in France and Italy, but interested instead in the history of institutions, notably hospitals; investigating the role of medicine in society rather than the intellectual pursuits of its leading practitioners.

Where scholars continued to take an interest in texts and in editing, they fell into two groups. The first was that of the classicists, concerned with fixing the manuscript base of their editions of ancient texts, principally Hippocrates, Dioscorides, and Galen. But these were Greek authors, and although familiar names in the Latin West, they wrote in Greek and, on the whole, their medieval Latin translations contributed little to the reestablishment of their original texts, particularly because the most influential texts of the time were translated into Latin from an Arabic translation of the original Greek. The one exception was the brilliant word-for-word versions of the South Italian, Niccolò da Reggio. Beloved of editors, his translations offered a way of regaining the very words of Galen, even if the Greek had been lost. But his translations, produced in the first half of the fourteenth century, came at a time when university courses were already standardized, and when few, even among the professors, bothered to read deeply into works that fell outside the curriculum.

The second modern group of medievalists concentrated on writings in the vernacular, particularly in English or German. They showed how the ideas of the learned physicians filtered down through society and how non-Latinate surgeons could develop their own sophisticated ideas on treatment. Recipe collections and short handbooks for the laity provided a bridge between elite and popular medicine.

Over the last thirty years there has been a revival in the study of medieval medicine. There have been major studies of medicine in Spain, Northern Italy, Paris, and England, to say nothing of a flood of controversial books on the Black Death. Textual studies have also flourished, not the least because of the linguistic interest in translations, particularly into Middle English. There have been regular conferences dedicated to Middle English texts, as well as to Latin medical texts from antiquity, with consequent publications of a variety of new material. Medicine pre-1000 AD in the Latin West has benefited from the researches of Klaus-Dietrich Fischer, among others, while codicologists and palaeographers have found many new texts in libraries both familiar and unfamiliar. Indeed, some of the more spectacular Latin finds have been made in the largest collections, where the disdain for, or unfamiliarity with, medieval medicine had frequently relegated manuscripts of this sort to the back of the queue for cataloguing. If one also considers the abundance of material now available online, from repertoires of manuscripts to photographs of the manuscripts themselves, the possibilities for scholarly progress in medieval medicine are enormous.

One must always remember, however, that a modern academic's understanding of medieval medical texts is likely to be very different from that of a medieval physician. The world of books, to say nothing of computers, is very different from that of manuscripts. That of abundant access to information fleetingly searched for minor queries can scarcely be compared to one in which a small number of texts were studied in enormous detail as the very foundations of a learned discipline. Few physicians in the Middle Ages, let alone their patients, possessed a library as full of relevant texts as a modern professor, and Latin, rather than their own vernacular, was the language of learning. Sources in Greek, Arabic, and Hebrew were inaccessible to all but a few, often aided by intermediaries with one or more of these languages as their native tongue. As a consequence, physicians had to rely on digests of various kinds to supplement the few texts at their disposal, some summarizing the essential points of Galenic doctrine, others providing a shortcut to therapeutic advice that had stood the test of generations, others creating short dictionaries for their own or others' use.

Despite their obvious significance, relatively little work has been done on these digests and repositories. Julius Pagel's editions of the dictionaries of two French physicians three generations apart, Johannes de Sancto Amando (1894) and Petrus de Sancto Floro (1896), are far from easy to use, even if modern technology has made them more accessible. Others, like Simon of Genoa, remain only in fallible printings from the Renaissance, a handicap to understanding the part they played in the transmission of medical knowledge around medieval Europe and, more importantly, from Classical Antiquity, via the Islamic world to the West.

The Simon of Genoa project, of which this volume forms a part, aims to provide a scholarly edition of his medical dictionary based on a collation of relevant manuscripts and early printed editions. The preliminary text, based on a 1510 printing, not only provides a more secure foundation for study, but also allows for a more precise investigation of his sources, which in turn may assist the editors of the texts and translations upon which Simon drew for his dictionary.

Sometimes, as in Valerie Knight's paper on Simon's use of the Latin Alexander of Tralles, one can come close to an identification of the actual manuscript, or at least manuscript family, on which he depended. Sometimes, as in Siam Bhayro's study of his use of Arabic sources, philology can throw light on the sort of Arabic that his Latin translator was using. Caroline Petit, in turn, focuses on Simon's use of a relatively rare portion of Galen, Book VI of his tract on simple drugs, to argue that he was using a Latin translation from the Arabic, and that, although there are copies of the original Greek text in circulation in Southern Italy, he did not take advantage of them. Indeed, as with Arabic, Simon's knowledge of the original language is far from clear, although he did know some Greek and he cites some unusual sources. More complex, as Marie Cronier shows, is his use of the Greek pharmacologist Dioscorides. In Simon's dictionary it is his description of plants that matters, not his assessment of their therapeutic properties. His sources for this author were almost certainly not directly Greek: both the references to a Greek codex and to illustrations in a Greek source are open to question, though that may not mean that he read widely into them. Instead, he relied largely on two different Latin translations, made at two different times. His main source is an arrangement of Dioscorides in alphabetical order, an obvious advantage for a dictionary writer, adapted from one of the three early Latin versions, the so-called 'Version C'. He also uses Version C itself, which is quite rare, but less frequently, and when he does, he often refers to it as being 'the real Dioscorides'. When his two sources conflict or fail, he has recourse to quotations in Latin from another tract ascribed to Dioscorides, *On feminine herbs*, which contains fragments taken from an even earlier Latin version, Version A, which he describes as coming from an 'old book'. Finally, he also makes use of quotations from Dioscorides in a text coming from Arabic, the so-called 'pseudo-Sarapion'. He himself may not have known Arabic to the extent of being able to read a long and complex book, but he seems to have set eyes on a copy of Dioscorides in Arabic with illustrations. Where he did so is unclear, but it is most likely to have been in Spain and the result of his friendship with the Jew Abraham of Tortosa. But although he gives a detailed description of what he saw, it cannot be easily reconciled with any existing manuscript. Similarly, his comments on a Greek illustrated manuscript do not fit the two major Greek manuscripts of this author that were in Southern Italy at this date. Analyzing his debt to authors closer in time is less difficult, simply because we can be sure that Simon had access to all the major Latin works of his day. As Charles Burnett shows, one of his main sources was the *Breviarium* of Stephen of Antioch, a digest of the new Arabic medicine in Latin dress.

Perhaps three quarters of Simon's entries in his dictionary deal with pharmacology, as Bouras-Vallianatos shows. His interest here is lexicographical rather than therapeutic, setting out a guide to what plants there are rather than analyzing their uses. This was not an easy task, because the variety of sources, not to mention the variety of languages on which they drew, was a source of confusion for centuries. The vagaries of medieval transmission only added to his difficulties, and his failure to always resolve them should not disguise his considerable talent in using and selecting the information at his disposal. The creation of a dictionary from what he had on hand was no easy feat.

Analyzing his sources is only the first stage in setting Simon in his intellectual context. He was a physician at the court of Pope Nicholas IV, and he had earlier collaborated with the Spanish Jew, Abraham of Tortosa, in the Latin translation of pseudo-Sarapion's *Liber aggregatus*. His origin in Genoa, a major Mediterranean trading city, would perhaps have brought him into contact with those who had visited Byzantium and the Greek settlements of Southern Italy, and it is perhaps from them that he derived his information on some Greek material that appears to be lost today. His papal connections would doubtless have also helped him, although at this stage the medical holdings of the papacy may not have been extensive or even accessible. His major conduit of information about Arabic sources is more likely to have been Spain than Sicily or the Maghreb.

As Peregrine Horden argues, our knowledge of Western medical culture, both inside and outside Rome at this date, is still far from complete, and it would be wrong to confine Simon's interests (and those of his fellow courtiers) solely to therapeutics. There were many new developments, from the provision of hospitals to autopsies. The growth of medical faculties in Italy and Southern France was just beginning and, though it was well established twenty or thirty years later, it was unclear which texts would be agreed upon to study. Although new Latin translations of Galen direct from Greek had been made, most doctors still relied on earlier versions, mainly from the Arabic, and on a handful of shorter texts that became known later as the *Articella*, The *Little art of medicine*. For therapeutics, the major sources were the great Arabic compendia that had been translated, mainly in Spain, during the early part of the century: Avicenna's *Canon* chief among them, as well as the older Salernitan Gariopontus. There was a fluidity in 1280 that was not there fifty years later.

But, educated though Simon was, with greater access to scholarly medicine than most of his contemporaries, he was no haunter of cloistered libraries. His dictionary reveals his activity as a traveller and his willingness to talk to the local inhabitants, at times in their own language. Some of his information on plants comes from conversing with Greeks, probably in Southern Italy, although both Genoa and Rome attracted traders from those regions. As Zipser points out, he seemed to have spoken with Arabic speakers in Spain, although whether he met the woman from Aleppo who told him the name of a plant there, or even on a visit to the Eastern Mediterranean, is not clear. What is obvious, however, is his willingness to gain knowledge from whatever source, without restricting himself to learned tomes, as well as his scrupulous recording of what he was told. He takes an unusual interest in the spelling and pronunciation of non-Latin words, sometimes so carefully that one may even detect regional dialects. His knowledge of plants in particular is not bound by the cover of his book.

Philology, as in these papers, serves a dual purpose: not only to present an accurate text but also to delineate the written sources that he used. Together they allow the historian to go further, and build up a picture of Simon as an educated man, as a traveller, and as a doctor. What he chose to include was only a selection of what he knew; chosen and organized for the benefit of his fellow doctors. One begins also to dimly see something of what he was; a good listener, an avid reader, and the sound organizer of a book that continued to be used for several more centuries to come.

Peregrine Horden

Medicine at the Papal Court in the Later Middle Ages: a Context for Simon of Genoa

Among the numerous works of the great thirteenth-century polymath, Ramon Llull, is the prose romance *Blanquerna*, which has some claim to be considered the first novel in European vernacular literature. Recounting how his eponymous hero becomes pope, Llull refers to 'un escriva en Arabic' at the papal curia, one of the great Christians of his age, seemingly a man with an international reputation for learning.[1] It is possible that Llull was referring to Simon of Genoa. If so, it is welcome testimony. We otherwise know very little about Simon beyond what he divulges in the preface to the *Clavis*. He held benefices in Padua and Rouen, and became subdeacon, chaplain, and personal physician to Pope Nicholas IV. He tells us that he travelled for almost thirty years gathering materials for his vast and magisterial glossary. He was still active in the early pontificate of Boniface VIII, completing his work before the death, in 1296, of Campano of Novara, whom he thanks in the preface. And that is virtually all we know of his biography.[2] The details of Simon's clerical career and intellectual development – including the real extent of his knowledge of Arabic – remain controversial.[3]

---

1 Agostino Paravicini-Bagliani, *Medicina e scienze della natura alla corte dei papi nel Duecento.* (Spoleto: Centro Italiano di Studi sull'Alto Medioevo, 1991), 184-5. It will be clear that I am heavily indebted throughout to this author's fundamental works on the thirteenth-century popes and the papal court (Agostino Paravicini-Bagliani, *Medicina e scienze della natura...*; *The Pope's Body*. Trans. by D. S. Peterson. (Chicago and London: University of Chicago Press, 2000), first published: *Il corpo del papa.* (Turin: Einaudi, 1994); *Il potere del papa: corporeità, autorappresentazione, simboli.* (Florence: Sismel/Galluzzo, 2009)), and differ from them only on minor points of emphasis and interpretation. I am also extremely grateful for advice and references to Charles Burnett, Jo Edge, Klaus-Dietrich Fischer, Monica Green, Vivian Nutton, Jennifer Rampling, Matthew Ross, Chris Wickham and Barbara Zipser. In what follows I have kept annotation to a minimum, just citing works that give full details of the people, texts and editions referred to. Names of historical figures have generally been Anglicized unless the original form is well known.

2 Paravicini-Bagliani, *Medicina e scienze della natura...*, 191-7, 247-51; *The Pope's Body*, 190-91.

3 For Simon's contact with Arabic speakers see Zipser, this volume; Bhayro, also this volume, takes a far dimmer view than did Llull of Simon's competence in the language. For the limited knowledge of Arabic at the papal court in Simon's time see Paravicini-Bagliani, *Medicina e scienze della natura...*, 180-81, 186-9.

So also do the circumstances in which the *Clavis* was commissioned and prepared. Was this work the fruit of Simon's own initiative or, as seems more likely, of papal patronage? What were his sources and where did he find them, and who helped him in the endeavour beyond the local informants to whom he occasionally refers? Although the *Simon Online* project to study the *Clavis* has identified thirty-seven or more of those sources, it is still not clear which libraries Simon used. Only one extant codex, the *Laurentian Celsus* (plut. 73,1),[4] can confidently be identified as a manuscript that he read – although it is also possible that one or other of two extant Spanish witnesses to an Arabic translation of Dioscorides were among his resources.[5]

Given the limited evidence available so far of Simon's career and his purposes, understanding of his work can advance on only two fronts. One is philological: close study of the *Clavis*, its analogues and possible sources. That is the approach of the other contributions in this collection. They focus on texts. The alternative, sketched here as a preliminary, is contextual and focuses on people: on the social history of medicine and doctors at the papal court, mainly but not exclusively in the long thirteenth century from the election of Innocent III to the death of Boniface VIII.[6]

*

The starting point must be this. The pope is a man – unless of course one credits the legend of Pope Joan, which became an ingredient in anti-papal polemic around the mid-thirteenth century, stressing, not coincidentally, the pontiff as physical, sexual, and of course, gendered being, with a desire for self-perpetuation.[7] The pope may be the 'Vicar of Christ', 'lower than God but higher than man', as Innocent III put it. The 'apex of the human race', he exercises *plenitudo potestatis*. Through the merits of St. Peter, of whom each pope is the direct heir, he is, in certain circumstances, *impeccabilis*, and thus well on the way to being infallible.[8]

---

4 Giuseppe Billanovich, "Centri di trasmissione: Milano, Nonantola, Brescia". In *La cultura antica nell' Occidente latino dal VII all' XI secolo*, I, (Spoleto: Presso la Sede del Centro, 1975), 328 n. 18. I owe this reference to Klaus-Dietrich Fischer.

5 See Cronier, this volume.

6 For detailed and accurate brief entries on all popes of the period see John N.D. Kelly, *The Oxford dictionary of popes*. (Oxford: Oxford University Press,1988).

7 Kelly, *The Oxford dictionary of popes*, appendix; Paravicini-Bagliani, *The Pope's Body*, 133.

8 Walter Ullmann, *The growth of papal government in the Middle Ages: a study in the ideological relation of clerical to lay power*. (London: Methuen, 1970); Brian Tierney, *Origins of papal infallibility, 1150-1350: a study on the concepts of infallibility, sovereignty and tradition in the Middle Ages*. (Leiden: Brill, 1972); Paravicini-Bagliani, *The Pope's Body*, 9-10.

Yet the pope is also a mere mortal, destined for a short reign.[9] 'Why does the head of the Apostolic See never live for very long but reaches his last day within a short space of time?' enquired Peter Damian in response to an enquiry from Alexander II (r. 1061–73); perturbed that none of his predecessors had survived for more than four or five years in office. Damian found no pontificate to have exceeded that traditionally attributed to St. Peter, that is, twenty-five years. Bernard of Clairvaux was well aware of this, just under a century later, when he wrote to Eugenius III (r. 1145–53): 'How many popes have you seen die in a just a short time? [...] the end of your office is not just certain but near'. 'Behold then two salutary ideas', Bernard further wrote, resuming the theme in his *De consideratione*: 'consider that you are the pope, and consider that you are – not that you were – a miserable speck of dust.' The return of dust to dust was likely to follow quite soon after consecration. There were twenty-seven or so popes (and one anti-pope) between Urban II and Boniface VIII whose year of birth is known or can be hazarded with some confidence.[10] Eleven were enthroned in their fifties, seven in their sixties, and eight in their seventies or eighties. The only outsider in this gerontocracy is Innocent III, a mere thirty-eight years old at his election. Even for him, St. Peter's twenty-five years might have seemed a far distant goal rather than a limitation. It is hardly surprising that no 'legitimate' pope surpassed that twenty-five year milestone until Pius IX in 1871.[11]

The tension between pope and speck of dust, between the exalted office and the frail mortal who held it, could be eased by separating the two out. The anonymous theorist of York, who (c. 1100) more or less invented the notion of the 'king's two bodies', went further with the pope and awarded him three bodies: supreme pontiff, above all men; human person, their equal; and sinful person, inferior to others, on a par with murderers and adulterers.[12]

✻

What attitude to medicine should such a tripartite figure take? St. Bernard would have known the answer. A pope, like a monk, he might have said, should not allow himself to be treated with anything more than common herbs, if that.[13] For Bernard, the opinions of Galen and Hippocrates were to be held in contempt.

---

9 For what follows see Paravicini-Bagliani, *The Pope's Body*, 11-13.

10 The figures that follow are based on data in Kelly, *The Oxford dictionary of Popes*.

11 Paravicini-Bagliani, *The Pope's Body*, 53.

12 *Ibidem*, 67.

13 Joseph Ziegler, *Medicine and religion c. 1300: the case of Arnau de Vilanova*. (Oxford: Clarendon Press, 1998), 219, 224.

Yet the papacy generally took a different view. Not many other pontiffs would have merited the criticism that the great Catalan physician Arnald of Villanova levelled at Boniface VIII, his most eminent patient: 'not zeal for Christ or health of souls ruled in him but [health] of bodies'.[14] Yet Boniface represents only one extreme of a spectrum – as Bernard represents the other. The pope, like any other mortal, was free to enjoy the benefit of secular medicine, provided – as enjoined by the Fourth Lateran Council (Canon 22) – he confessed his sins first and put the medicine of the soul above that of the body. Hippocrates and Galen were portrayed in the cathedral crypt at Anagni, probably at the behest of the canons there. These men, in turn, were closely connected with Innocent III and still more Gregory IX, under whom the court often moved to Viterbo for the summer.[15] The Augustinian theologian James of Viterbo (c.1255–c.1308) even opined that medicine would have been useful in Paradise, before sin, and thus sickness, arose.[16] After all, the doctor's skill and means of curing alike came from God (*Ecclesiasticus* 38.1–4). Canon law restricted the practice of medicine only by those in major orders and living under a rule and was meant to deter them from practising it for profit.[17] Hence, for example, over a third of the practitioners known from medieval France (between the twelfth and fifteenth centuries) were members of the clergy.[18]

Broken down by century, that proportion was probably at its highest in the twelfth century and started to decline in the thirteenth. In 1219 Honorius III extended the scope of the prohibition from those living under a rule to a wider array of archdeacons, deacons, rural deans, and others holding benefices, and also to priests. But the measure was intended to protect the study of theology and was directed at medical learning more than at medical practice.[19] Even Celestine V, who tried to prevent all clerics from practising medicine, exempted those whose cures were administered to family and friends or to others free, out of charity. Dispensations from all these measures could in any case be secured, and the measures' scope was soon reduced, essentially so that parish clergy were untouched by the canon law on this matter; reduced by – predictably – Boniface VIII. The exempted included – the very tip of the clerical-medical iceberg – those major figures such as Teodorico Borgognoni, the surgeon who became a bishop, and above all Peter of Spain. Unless two distinct figures are being conflated by

---

14 Paravicini-Bagliani, *The Pope's Body*, 227.
15 *Ibidem*, 178, 187.
16 Ziegler, *Medicine and religion c. 1300*, 201-2.
17 Darrel W. Amundsen, *Medicine, society, and faith in the ancient and medieval worlds.* (Baltimore and London: Johns Hopkins University Press, 1996), 227-35.
18 Ziegler, *Medicine and religion c. 1300*, 3.
19 Amundsen, *Medicine, society, and faith...*, 231-3.

historians, Peter, who began as Dean of Lisbon, perhaps went on to serve as personal physician to Gregory X (of which clear evidence is lacking), became archbishop of Braga, and finally, having been made Cardinal, was elected pope as John XXI in 1276.[20]

With such a progression possible, it is hardly remarkable that leading abbots and bishops should retain doctors, or that the papal court should attract and welcome many of them. The unsurpassed scholarship of Paravicini-Bagliani has given us a detailed prosopography of over seventy medical men known or conjectured to have some association with popes and cardinals during the long twelfth century.[21] The list is 'end heavy': more than a third of them (twenty-five) were active under Boniface VIII, other pontificates variously attracting only up to six names. Those who may have been specifically papal physicians range in number between one and three per reign, but again the tally rises under Boniface, to five. As with papal chaplains (who are being studied by Matthew Ross of University College, London), some associations between medical men and popes or cardinals are transient and ad hoc while some are very lasting. According to the Renaissance chronicler Filippo Villani, Taddeo Alderotti cured Honorius IV of some ailment but that was his only recorded connection with the curia and it may not even be historical. At the other end of the spectrum, Campano of Novarra was active for some thirty years at court under four popes, from Urban IV to Boniface VIII, and William of Brescia served Boniface VII, Clement V, and John XXII.

These examples immediately indicate that many of the names involved are major figures in the general history of scholarly medicine in the period. To the list we can probably add Philip of Tripoli, Richard of Fournival, Teodorico Borgognoni, William of Moerbeke, Arnald of Villanova (Arnald perhaps the most significant for European medicine as a whole in this roster of luminaries), and of course, not least, Simon of Genoa. The papal court was obviously an attractive source of patronage. We note the interplay of medical and clerical careers, medical success leading to clerical preferment as with Teodorico Borgognoni who probably rose to be papal penitentiary and chaplain on the strength of having cured Innocent IV's nephew. Campano of Novara clearly became very rich during his long service as astronomer/astrologer as well as doctor at the curia. He had a palace in Viterbo and his landed wealth was appraised at more than twelve thousand florins.[22] Paravicini-Bagliani's study of cardinals' wills shows

---

20 Paravicini-Bagliani, *Medicina e scienze della natura...*, 28-9, 32.

21 Unless otherwise indicated, all details of papal doctors in the following paragraphs derive from Paravicini-Bagliani, *Medicina e scienze della natura...*, 3-51.

22 Paravicini-Bagliani, *The Pope's Body*, 189.

more generally that their bequests to personal physicians usually outstripped in generosity those to other *familiares*.[23] The rewards of service could take a variety of forms. Richard of Fournival was dispensed from the restriction of canon law so that he could practise surgery, as presumably at some point was Teodorico. Richard of Wendover (who may or may not be the same as Richard the Englishman) received an ivory cross from Gregory IX on his death-bed. Arnald of Villanova was given a gold cross by Boniface VIII. John of Procida gained political intercession over some property in Naples that he had lost by backing the wrong horse in the imperial succession dispute. His patient, a cardinal and future pope, wrote to the current pope, Clement IV, asking him to intercede with Charles of Anjou.[24]

In the first half of the thirteenth century a substantial number of papal medical men may have been educated at Salerno, for example the cardinal John of St. Paul.[25] This connection weakens in the second half of the century, as doctors seem more likely to have come from cities in the Papal States. By the end of the century, perhaps from the 1280s, there may have been some teaching of medicine in the *Studium curiae*, and this could have provided an alternative reservoir of skill and talent.[26]

One sign of the growing general esteem for medicine on the part of the thirteenth-century papacy is that doctors seem to become an indispensable presence at the pope's death-bed. Another is that the remedies that doctors were believed, rightly or not, to have created for popes were celebrated as such in the wider manuscript literature of medical procedures. Albertus Magnus was never a curial physician so far as is known, but that did not hinder the transmission of the *pillule mirabilis operationis* that he is credited with having made for Gregory IX.[27]

*

Some caveats need mentioning, none the less. Paravicini-Bagliani's prosopography, though of impeccable scholarship and wholly indispensable, is full of conjectural identifications, not least that of Peter of Spain and Pope John XXI. This is inevitable given the state of the evidence, and the author

---

23 Paravicini-Bagliani, *The Pope's Body*, 191; *I testamenti dei cardinali del Duecento*. (Rome: Presso la Società, 1980).

24 Paravicini-Bagliani, *The Pope's Body*, 191.

25 Paravicini-Bagliani, *Il potere del papa...*, 97-112.

26 But the evidence is controversial and the details obscure: Paravicini-Bagliani, *Medicina e scienze della natura...*, 393-408.

27 *Ibidem*, 7-8, 21-2, 24, 27, 49.

never disguises the fact. But it is still worth occasionally questioning the criteria of inclusion. Romuald very probably did become archbishop of Salerno, for example, but should he be listed as a doctor at the papal court on the strength of a line of verse by Giles of Corbeil saying he was admired by the curia as a medical writer and a 'patron of life'? Or again was Innocent III's doctor, Romanus, the same as the cardinal bishop whose sole recorded claim to medical expertise is his awareness of the rather basic notion that medicine heals by contraries? Should Adam of Kircudbright, chaplain to Urban IV, be listed when his medical fame is reportedly that he served as Robert the Bruce's doctor? Peter of Abano dedicated a treatise on poisons to a pope but we cannot tell which one; and although he claimed to enjoy papal favour it is not clear that he practised at the curia either.

We can pick out individual pieces of the jigsaw and show that they do not quite fit together. But the overall picture is still robust enough to convey the substantial presence of authorities on medical practice in and near the papal court. And that provides some context for Simon. In this medical activity he was one of many. He blends into the crowd of doctors clustering round popes and cardinals hoping for medical patronage and ecclesiastical preferment. In the longevity of his association with the curia he was unusual but by no means unique.

For us, however, Simon is known as a text more than as a person; and on this front too, it is possible to sketch a context within which his decades of work on the *Clavis* come to seem, not less remarkable, but at least a little more explicable. This is not the place for detail; but again from the fundamental work of Paravicini-Bagliani, it is clear that during the thirteenth century the papal court was increasingly a focus for a number of scientific interests – scientific in both the medieval and the modern senses.[28] Astronomy and geometry (Campano of Novarra), geography (David of Dinant), and optics are only some of the subjects read or written about at court. The concentration of expertise could be unrivalled: 'in the decade 1267–77, Viterbo was the European capital of optics'.[29] That is thanks to the intersection, in the papal ambit, of the careers of William of Moerbeke, Witelo, John Peckham, and Peter of Spain, at Viterbo in the Papal States, where the curia resided almost without interruption from 1260 to 1280.[30]

Medical writings, too, belong under this heading of scientific patronage. To give only the main topics and some key names associated with each in the curial world:[31] surgery (Teodorico), anatomy (David of Dinant again), nutrition

---

28 For what follows see *Ibidem*, 14, 16, 23-4, 42, 48, 87-115, 119-24, 143-75, 161-5.
29 Paravicini-Bagliani, *The Pope's Body*, 196–7, 209.
30 *Ibidem*, 173.
31 Paravicini-Bagliani, *Medicina e scienze della natura*, 13, 16, 25, 32, 41-2.

(at Viterbo William of Moerbeke translated Galen on this, as later, in Rome, did Accursino of Pistoia), and regimen (John of Toledo, John of Capua, Peter of Spain, and most notably Arnald, whom Boniface more or less immured in a papal castle in order to focus his mind on the task of writing a regimen for him). Surgery, anatomy, nutrition, regimen – these are topics in standard Galenic medicine of the period. But the papal court became a centre for speculation and writing about less predictable, even occult, topics. One of them was the question of how to delay the ill effects of old age and to prolong life. Instead of being cut short like St. Peter, might the pope instead outdo Peter and even rival Methuselah? Involved here were alchemical remedies. It is no coincidence that Philip of Tripoli translated at the curia the pseudo-Aristotelian *Secreta secretorum* (*Secret of Secrets*).[32] Besides devoting considerable space to prolongation of life, this text, the most widely read 'Aristotelian' title of the Middle Ages, was a source for much of the thinking about alchemy, physiognomy, magic, and astrology of the thirteenth to fourteenth centuries. Those who insinuated that Peter of Spain/John XXI died suddenly despite boasting that he could prolong his life, presumably with an elixir, or that several cardinals quaffed potable gold, may have known more than we do about the extent and the seriousness of curial interest in alchemy.[33]

Simon and his *Clavis* can to some extent be understood against this background. For example, it is clear that he consulted alchemical treatises.[34] Yet he also stands out because of the magnitude of the task he set himself and the time he took to complete it. In this context the analogy with Witelo's work on optics and Campano's on Euclid or on the planets may be just as relevant. Both scholars were committed to major synoptic undertakings. Perhaps Simon was aiming for a similar comprehensiveness.[35]

＊

Why such a comprehensive approach? Why all the scientific and medical activity that fed into it? Why was the papal court a centre of patronage on this scale? Paravicini-Bagliani's answer, given at several points in his more

---

32 Steven Williams, *The Secret of Secrets: the scholarly career of a pseudo-Aristotelian text in the later Middle Ages.* (Ann Arbor: University of Michigan Press, 2003), 114-21.

33 Paravicini-Bagliani, *The Pope's Body*, 210-11. For continuing curial interest in alchemy see also 221, 249, 346n., with Chiara Crisciani, *Il papa e l'alchemia: Felice V, Guglielmo Fabri e l'elixir.* (Rome: Viella, 2002).

34 See *Clavis* entries for *Elcismatos, Muzadir,* and *Sponium,* to which Barbara Zipser kindly directed my attention.

35 I am indebted here to Charles Burnett.

recent work,[36] is simple: the impact of the new knowledge becoming available as Arabic texts were translated. The translation activity and the reception of learning in Arabic, especially works of Aristotle and Avicenna, can be documented quite amply at the thirteenth-century curia.[37] That fact is not self-explanatory. Such texts do not arrive of their own accord. They have to be identified as desirable and sought out, and then laboriously translated. If we see the various forms of exoteric and esoteric learning in which popes and cardinals of our period took some interest as merely reflex responses to a new fashion in philosophical medicine, we miss the sense of excitement, the fervour of the hunt for new therapeutic possibilities, that news of the latter engendered. Aged and decrepit cardinals, and still more popes, living (some of the time, when unavoidable) in a notoriously insalubrious city, had many reasons to encourage novel ideas and techniques. Aspiring curialist doctors had many reasons to offer such novelties. In other words, the explanation of the texts is to be sought in the history of the patients involved; it is not that the arrival of the texts explains the attitudes and enthusiasms of the patients.

This is by no means to deny that wider contexts may also have had some bearing. Interaction with, and emulation of, the imperial court of Frederick II should not be discounted.[38] Nor should we forget that this century of natural philosophy, of 'scientific' celebration and investigation of the material world, was also the century of Catharism, with its denigration of that world: a heresy as evident in the Papal States as it was in the Languedoc, and slow to succumb to the Inquisition.[39] Yet such wider concerns will have seemed secondary to Gregory IX, with his gallstones, or to Honorius IV, so crippled by gout that he needed a crutch for support when celebrating mass.[40]

There was nothing very new about this. Paravicini-Bagliani treats his long thirteenth century as a self-contained period. For him, it begins in clear-cut fashion with Innocent III, the first pope for whom we know of a *medicus pape*; the first pope to have discussed his own maladies at some length; the first pope to have acquired a house for his doctor near the Vatican palace.[41] These claims for outright novelty on Innocent's behalf would have surprised many of his predecessors. Popes had been consulting the most learned doctors

---

36 e.g. Paravicini-Bagliani, *The Pope's Body*, XIV, 185.

37 For Simon's use of Arabic manuscripts see Cronier, this volume; Paravicini-Bagliani, *Medicina e scienze della natura...*, 179-232.

38 Paravicini-Bagliani, *Medicina e scienze della natura...*, XIII, 55-84.

39 Roger Kenneth French, Andrew Cunningham, *Before science: the invention of the friars' natural philosophy*. (Aldershot: Scolar, 1996).

40 Paravicini-Bagliani, *The Pope's Body*, 183, 194.

41 *Ibidem*, 186-7.

they could find since the time of Gregory the Great in the late sixth century if not earlier.[42] Of course there were changes of scale. Chris Wickham's personal database of charters and documentary evidence, compiled as part of a project and forthcoming monograph on Rome and its environs, 900–1200 (the period before that of Paravicini-Bagliani), finds some thirty-two medical men for the whole three centuries. That seems a small number in comparison, even though the database excludes narratives, which would surely yield more names. Yet it is not clear that changes in quality as well as quantity were under way as we move into the thirteenth century. Is a *medicus pape* necessarily more than a doctor who attends the pope, even if he lives in a 'tied cottage'; or has he moved into a new category of 'papal physician'? The Latin is ambiguous. Granted, in the thirteenth century the credentials that an aspiring doctor derived from acquaintance with the new Arabic-derived learning would have made some difference. But we need to ask: what sort of medicine was regularly dispensed to aging pontiffs and their courtiers? Was it elixirs of life or something more basic? For evidence we have to look forward a little into the Avignon period, where the comings and goings of doctors at the curia can be documented in a similar way.[43] And to get a little nearer to the papal sickbed in that period we can sometimes turn to catalogues of *experimenta* – tried and tested remedies, rather than experiments in the modern sense, but 'experimental' in that no one knew how or why they worked. Their claim to repeated use lay in their effectiveness.

Arnald of Villanova recorded seventy-three successful 'experimental' treatments that he conducted on named individuals at or around the papal court in Avignon between 1305 and 1311.[44] Although the treatments include use of gems, gold, mercury, and alcohol, Arnald's remedies depend mostly on vegetable ingredients, and are simple – far more so than those he expounded (to impress colleagues or patrons?) in many of his theoretical works. And some of the ailments he addresses (in patients of both sexes) hardly seem worthy of the foremost 'consultant' of his time. They include haemorrhoids, wrinkles, hair loss, and fleas, as well as amnesia, chronic headaches, indigestion, swellings, and toothaches.

---

42 Peregrine Horden, "The late antique origins of the lunatic asylum?" In Philip Rousseau, Emmanuel Papoutsakis (Eds.), *Transformations of late antiquity: essays for Peter Brown*. (Farnham: Ashgate, 2009), 265.

43 Paul Pansier, "Les médecins des papes d'Avignon (1308–1403)". *Janus* 14 (1909): 405-34; Bernard Guillemain, *La cour pontificale d'Avignon (1309–1376): Étude d'une société.* (Paris: de Boccard, 1962).

44 Michael McVaugh, "The *Experimenta* of Arnald of Villanova". *Journal of Medieval and Renaissance Studies* 1 (1971): 107–18.

Another *experimentum* for toothache. Once the lord pope [Clement V, the collection's dedicatee] had a pain in his jaw [...] One of his teeth had a cavity and there a worm tossed to and fro. When the worm stirred within the tooth the aforementioned lord suffered greatly, so that he could neither drink nor sleep. After I had carefully inspected it, I easily administered a remedy [...] I caused to be gathered a certain herb called chamomile in the vernacular.[45]

Arnald fumigated the pontiff's mouth with smoke from heated chamomile seeds and the worm dropped out. If this is generally what we would have found at the pope's bedside, it may come as a surprise after all the arcane learning with which the court has been associated. But it would not have surprised twelfth-century physicians. There may be more continuity between twelfth and thirteenth centuries than Paravicini-Bagliani supposes; and that continuity too would be a further part of the explanation for the medical history of the curia during the period in which Simon was active. There was a more long-standing tradition of medical patronage behind it.

*

'Try anything once – or, indeed, repeatedly', might have been the unofficial papal motto where health and illness were concerned. *Experimenta* and basic herbal remedies at one end of the spectrum: the most recherché alchemical techniques at the other. One clear example of this 'no holds barred' approach is the frequency with which popes of the later Avignon period, the Great Schism, and after, happily resorted to Jewish doctors (as did archbishops, bishops, abbots, and priests below them).[46] Hebrew sources alone claim that Master Gaio (Isaac ben Mordecai) served as doctor to Nicholas IV, and that seems too early by comparison with the plentiful evidence from later on. But Boniface IX, for example, had two Jewish physicians in attendance. Such men were educated and skilful, and they were available in abundance, for this was a period when, following the various expulsions from northern kingdoms, the concentration of Jewish doctors in Provence and adjacent regions was at its greatest.

---

45 McVaugh, "The *Experimenta* of Arnald of Villanova", 113; trans. Faith Wallis, *Medieval medicine: a reader*. (Toronto: University of Toronto Press, 2010), 402.

46 For what follows see Joseph Shatzmiller, *Jews, medicine, and medieval society*. (Berkeley and London: University of California Press, 1994), 94-5, and Nancy Siraisi, *Medieval and early Renaissance medicine*. (Chicago and London: University of Chicago Press, 1990), 29. See further Anna Esposito, "Alla corte dei Papi: archiatri pontifici ebrei tra '400 e '500." in Elisa Andretta, Marilyn Nicoud (Eds.), *Être médecin à la cour (Italie, France, Espagne, XIIIe–XVIIIe siècle)*. (Florence: Sismel/Galuzzo, 2013), 17–33. This important volume appeared while the present collection was already in press.

If all else fails, try magic. Papal magic seems to belong under the heading of the slanders and trumped-up charges levelled, at various points in the later Middle Ages and Renaissance, against popes and anti-popes alike. But there is more to the subject. Popes in earlier periods wore apotropaic bells attached to the hem of their vestments.[47] At his posthumous trial, Boniface VIII was alleged to have received an *idolum* containing a diabolical spirit from Taddeo Alderotti.[48] Yet it is likely that Arnald of Villanova really did present the same pope with a talisman in the form of a gold seal for use against his kidney stones.[49] Around 1315 the future pope Clement VI copied out an illicit form of divination by name (onomancy).[50] In 1318, John XXII fulminated against a network of spirit conjurors in a letter, but was frank about the fact that they included several people residing at his own court.[51] And so on. Later, the genuine interest of Benedict XIII and his circle in alchemy, astrology, and Joachimite prophecy could have provided the kernel for the fantastic charges of witchcraft and necromancy brought against him at the Council of Pisa in 1409.[52]

*

The history of the connections between popes and medicine in the long thirteenth century (the century when papal monarchy was at its apogee) could be pursued further in many directions: for example: hospital foundation, the medicalizing of canonization procedures, concern with autopsy and dissection, and with division of the corpse for burial.[53] None of these, though, would shed particular light on Simon of Genoa and his *Clavis*. We can try to set him in a wider curial context and a longer history of papal patronage of science and medicine. Yet he remains an elusive figure, whose work we are only just beginning to understand.

---

47 Henry Maguire, "Magic and money in the early Middle Ages". *Speculum* 72 (4) (1997): 1038-9.

48 Paravicini-Bagliani, *Medicina e scienze della natura...*, 36.

49 Michael McVaugh, *Medicine before the Plague: practitioners and their patients in the Crown of Aragon 1285–1345.* (Cambridge: Cambridge University Press, 1993), 162-3.

50 Jean-Patrice Boudet, *Entre science et nigromancie: astrologie, divination et magie dans l'Occident médiéval.* (Paris: Sorbonne, 2006), 43. A reference I owe to Jo Edge.

51 Peter George Maxwell-Stuart, (Ed. and trans.) *The occult in medieval Europe, 500–1500.* (Houndmills: Palgrave Macmillan, 2005), 84-6. For wider context see Alain Boureau, *Satan the heretic: the birth of demonology in the medieval West.* (Chicago: University of Chicago Press, 2000).

52 Margaret Harvey, "Papal witchcraft: the charges against Benedict XIII". In Derek Baker (ed.), *Sanctity and Secularity: the Church and the world* (Oxford: Ecclesiastical History Society, 1973), 109-16.

53 See e.g. Debra Birch, *Pilgrimage to Rome in the Middle Ages.* (Woodbridge: Boydell, 1998), 141-3; Joseph Ziegler, 'Practitioners and saints: medical men and canonization procedures in the thirteenth to fifteenth centuries'. *Social History of Medicine* 12 (2), (1999): 191-225; Katharine Park *Secrets of women: gender, generation, and the origins of human dissection.* (New York: Zone, 2006), 47, 52.

Bibliography

Amundsen, Darrel W. *Medicine, society, and faith in the ancient and medieval worlds*. Baltimore and London: Johns Hopkins University Press, 1996.

Billanovich, Giuseppe. "Centri di trasmissione: Milano, Nonantola, Brescia." In *La cultura antica nell' Occidente latino dal VII all' XI secolo*, I, Spoleto: Presso la Sede del Centro, 1975.

Birch, Debra. *Pilgrimage to Rome in the Middle Ages*. Woodbridge: Boydell, 1998.

Boudet, Jean-Patrice. *Entre science et nigromancie: astrologie, divination et magie dans l'Occident médiéval*. Paris: Sorbonne, 2006.

Boureau, Alain. *Satan the heretic: the birth of demonology in the medieval West*. Chicago: University of Chicago Press, 2006.

Crisciani, Chiara. *Il papa e l'alchemia: Felice V, Guglielmo Fabri e l'elixir*. Rome: Viella, 2002.

Esposito, Anna. "Alla corte dei Papi: archiatri pontifici ebrei tra '400 e '500." In Elisa Andretta, Marilyn Nicoud (Eds.), *Être médecin à la cour (Italie, France, Espagne, XIIIe–XVIIIe siècle)*. 17–33. Florence: Sismel/Galuzzo, 2013.

French, Roger K. and Andrew Cunningham. *Before science: the invention of the friars' natural philosophy*. Aldershot: Scolar, 1996.

Guillemain, Bernard. *La cour pontificale d'Avignon (1309–1376): Étude d'une société*. Paris: de Boccard, 1962.

Harvey, Margaret. "Papal witchcraft: the charges against Benedict XIII." In *Sanctity and Secularity: the Church and the world.* edited by D. Baker, 109-16. Oxford: Ecclesiastical History Society, 1973.

Horden, Peregrine, "The late antique origins of the lunatic asylum?" In *Transformations of late antiquity: essays for Peter Brown.* edited by Philip Rousseau and Emmanuel Papoutsakis, 259-78. Farnham: Ashgate, 2009.

Kelly, John N. D. *The Oxford Dictionary of Popes.* Oxford: Oxford University Press, 1988.

Maguire, Henry. "Magic and money in the early Middle Ages." *Speculum* 72 no.4 (1997): 1037-54.

Maxwell-Stuart, Peter G., ed. and trans. *The occult in medieval Europe, 500–1500.* Houndmills: Palgrave Macmillan, 2005.

McVaugh, Michael, "The *Experimenta* of Arnald of Villanova." *Journal of Medieval and Renaissance Studies* 1 (1971): 107–18.

— *Medicine before the Plague: practitioners and their patients in the Crown of Aragon 1285–1345.* Cambridge: Cambridge University Press, 1993.

Pansier, Pierre. "Les médecins des papes d'Avignon (1308–1403)." *Janus* 14 (1909): 405-34.

Paravicini-Bagliani, Agostino. *I testamenti dei cardinali del Duecento.* Rome: Presso la Società, 1980.

— *Medicina e scienze della natura alla corte dei papi nel Duecento.* Spoleto: Centro Italiano di Studi sull'Alto Medioevo, 1991.

— *The Pope's Body.* Transated by David S. Peterson. Chicago and London: University of Chicago Press (first published 1994. *Il corpo del papa.* Turin: Einaudi), 2000.

— *Il potere del papa: corporeità, autorappresentazione, simboli.* Florence: Sismel/ Galluzzo, 2009.

Park, Katharine. *Secrets of women: gender, generation, and the origins of human dissection.* New York: Zone, 2006.

Shatzmiller, Joseph. *Jews, medicine, and medieval society.* Berkeley and London: University of California Press, 1994.

Siraisi, Nancy G. *Medieval and early Renaissance medicine.* Chicago and London: University of Chicago Press, 1990.

Tierney, Brian. *Origins of papal infallibility, 1150-1350: a study on the concepts of infallibility, sovereignty and tradition in the Middle Ages.* Leiden: Brill, 1972.

Ullmann, Walter. *The growth of papal government in the Middle Ages: a study in the ideological relation of clerical to lay power.* London: Methuen, 1970.

Wallis, Faith ed. *Medieval medicine: a reader.* Toronto: University of Toronto Press, 2010.

Williams, Steven J. *The 'Secret of secrets': the scholarly career of a pseudo-Aristotelian text in the later Middle Ages.* Ann Arbor: University of Michigan Press, 2003.

Ziegler, Joseph. *Medicine and religion c. 1300: the case of Arnau de Vilanova.* Oxford: Clarendon Press, 1998.

— "Practitioners and saints: medical men and canonization procedures in the thirteenth to fifteenth centuries." *Social History of Medicine* 12 no 2 (1999): 191-225.

— "Medicine and immortality in terrestrial paradise." In *Religion and medicine in the Middle Ages.* edited by Peter Biller and Joseph Ziegler, 201-42. York: York Medieval Press, 2001.

Edited by **Barbara Zipser**

Petros Bouras-Vallianatos (King's College London)

Simon of Genoa's *Clavis sanationis*: a Study of Thirteenth-Century Latin Pharmacological Lexicography.[1]

Introduction

In the course of the thirteenth century, medieval medicine was in the process of adapting and evaluating certain elements recently introduced by the twelfth-century Latin translations of Arabic and Greek works.[2] Although some of the early translators attempted to eliminate foreign words from their works, at other times new terms were invented by simply transliterating Arabic words into Latin. Moreover, forgotten Classical Greek terms, that had been preserved by Islamic authors, now reappeared.[3] At the same time, after the fall of Constantinople to the Crusaders in 1204 and the creation of various Western principalities in Greece and the Middle East, there was a consequent influx of Westerners to the East. This stimulated the exchange of ideas and developed the interrelationships between East and West, which resulted in the circulation of Greek and Arabic medical texts, often previously unknown to Western scholars.[4] Thus, a vast number of new terms and details on various aspects of medicine from ophthalmology to

---

1 I am grateful to Charles Burnett, Vivian Nutton, and Barbara Zipser for their comments on the paper I delivered at the conference, and, in particular, to Dionysios Stathakopoulos, for his advice and suggestions on a later draft.

2 For an introduction to the 12th-c. translators, see Marie-Thérèse d'Alverny, "Translations and Translators". In Robert L. Benson and Giles Constable (Eds.), *Renaissance and Renewal in the Twelfth Century,* (Cambridge: Harvard University Press, 1982), 421-462.

3 See Gotthard Strohmaier, "Constantine's pseudo-Classical terminology and its survival." In Charles Burnett and Danielle Jacquart (Eds.), *Constantine the African and 'Alī Ibn al-'Abbās al-Maǧdūsī* (Leiden: Brill, 1994), 90-98.

4 For example, Peter of Abano (c. 1250–c. 1315), philosopher and professor of medicine in Padua, sojourned in Constantinople at some time between 1270 and 1290 in order to investigate Greek medical manuscripts; see Paolo Marangon, "Per una revisione cell'interpretazione di Pietro d'Abano". In Paolo Marangon (Ed.), *Il pensiero ereticale nella Marca Trevigiana e a Venezia dal 1200 al 1350* (Abano Terme, Padova: Francisci 1984), 66-104. On Peter's Latin translations of Galen, see Lynn Thorncike, "Translations of Works of Galen from the Greek by Peter of Abano". *Isis* 33 (1942), 649-653; and Stefania Fortuna, "Pietro d'Abano e le traduzioni Latine di Galeno". *Medicina nei Secoli,* 20 (2008): 447-463.

surgery and pharmacology, previously unexplored or little discussed, were now available. In particular, in the field of pharmacy, the separation of the profession of physician from that of apothecary by an edict of the Holy Roman Emperor Frederick II (1220 – 1250) promulgated sometime between 1231 and 1240, confirms the concern at the time for the provision of well-researched and well-prepared medicaments.[5]

Two main categories of texts, connected with the identification of various pharmacological ingredients and the preparation of drugs, were available at that time in the West. Firstly, there are alphabetical books of simples, with the various versions of the work of Dioscorides (fl. AD 65) foremost among them.[6] The various herbals usually derived from earlier Dioscorides manuscripts, come into the same category; these books with their colorful illustrations constitute the most important tool for the identification of various plant-based ingredients.[7] Related to the texts devoted to simples mentioned above, there are also lists of compound drugs called *antidotaria*. Such texts are usually arranged alphabetically in accordance with the type of compound, i.e. oils, ointments, powders, collyria, purgatives, etc.[8] The second category includes works with titles such as: *glossaria*, *hermeneumata*, *synonyma*, etc.[9] These texts provide lists of technical terms in alphabetical order with the formula *id est* followed by the corresponding Latin

---

5 The edict was not an isolated legislative act, but part of Frederick II's legislation issued with a view to controlling hygiene regulations in Southern Italy; cf. Wolfgang-Hagen Hein, Kurt Sappert, *Die Medizinalordnung Friedrichs: Eine pharmaziehistorische Studie.* (Eutin: Internationale Gesellschaft für Geschichte der Pharmazie, 1957), 17-18 and 98.

6 The *Alphabetical Dioscorides* was the most widespread version between the early 12th-c. and the late 15th-c.; see John M. Riddle, "The Latin Alphabetical Dioscorides Manuscript Group." *Proceedings of the XIIIth International Congress for the History of Science, Acts Section IV,* (1974), 204-209.

7 See Minta Collins, *Medieval Herbals.* (London: British Library and University of Toronto, 2000), 153-220 and 307-308, who describes and discusses the function of different versions of 12th- and 13th-c. Latin herbal compilations.

8 The earliest and most widespread Western collection of compounds was the 12th-c. *Antidotarium Nicolai*, which seems to have been compiled in Salerno; see Gundolf Keil, "Zur Datierung des *Antidotarium Nicolai*." *Sudhoffs Archiv* 62 (1978): 190-6. See also Dietlinde Goltz, *Mittelalterliche Pharmazie und Medizin. Dargestellt an Geschichte und Inhalt des Antidotarium Nicolai.* (Stuttgart: Wissenschaftliche Verlagsgesellschaft, 1976), who discusses the work in the light of contemporary medicine and pharmacy.

9 See MacKinney, who explains the nature and function of medieval medical glossaries and dictionaries. (Loren C. MacKinney, "Medieval medical dictionaries and glossaries." In Lea James Cate, Eugene Anderson (Eds.), *Medieval historiographical essay: in honor of James Westfall Thompson.* (Chicago: The University of Chicago Press, 1938), 240-268). For a fresh description and comparison of the medieval glossaries in connection with the *Synonyma alphita*, see Alejandro García González, *Alphita*. (Firenze: SISMEL edizioni del Galluzzo, 2008), 8-21 and 71-86.

or vernacular word.[10] A vast number of their entries are related to pharmacology, mentioning various substances.[11] Finally, there are numerous other texts of the same nature, which were composed particularly as handbooks to facilitate the reading of the recent Latin translations of Islamic authors.[12]

It is quite evident that in parallel with the great activity in the area of translation and revision of Classical works, considerable efforts were made in the field of lexicography. MacKinney, emphasizing the extraordinary number of such works, aptly states that 'during the early Middle Ages [...] it was the epitomizers and lexicographers who held the center of the stage.'[13] Simon of Genoa, however, in contrast to other thirteenth-century authors, makes a considerable advance in composing a comprehensive, updated work, the *Clavis sanationis*, which could be considered a medical dictionary rather than simply a glossary. The work consists of 6,500 entries in alphabetical order and is substantiated by Simon's own comments. This paper presents a study of the pharmacological sections of the *Clavis sanationis* focusing on and interpreting various categories of the data provided, but also exploring their practical value. As I would like to demonstrate below, the work could be seen as a substantial response to contemporary needs, providing apothecaries and physicians with essential details.

Simon's Life and the Thirteenth-Century Papal Court

There is little biographical data for Simon of Genoa's life. From the incipit of his *Clavis* we can deduce that Simon was a member of the papal curia of Pope Nicholas IV (1288–1292), serving as *subdyaconus* and *capellanus medicus*.[14]

---

10 One of the earliest texts of such kind is the *Synonyma alphita*, a glossary of probably Salernitan origin, which consists of 1269 entries and seems to have been written before 1250. For a new edition and commentary, see González, *Alphita*, 139-575.

11 For example, in the *Synonyma alphita* almost half of the entries, 57%, are dedicated to the interpretation of medicinal plants; *Ibidem*, 25-28.

12 For example the *Synonyma Rasis* and those for the works of Serapion, Avicenna, Haly Abbas etc. For a discussion of various handbooks with synonyms for words used by Islamic authors, see Danielle Jacquart, "Arabisants du Moyen Age et de la Renaissance: Jérôme Ramusio († 1486) correcteur de Gérard de Crémone († 1187)." *Bibliothèque de l'École des Chartes* 147 (1989): 407-408; and Danielle Jacquart and Françoise Micheau, *La médecine arabe et l'Occident médiéval*. (Paris: Maissonneuve et Larose, 1990), 163-164.

13 MacKinney "Medieval medical dictionaries and glossaries", 267.

14 Quotations of Simon's *Clavis sanationis* follow the online transcription in *Simon Online* at http://www.simonofgenoa.org. *Clavis*, Incipit: '*Incipit clavis sanationis elaborate per venerabilem virum magistrum Simonem Ianuensem domini pape subdyaconum et capellanum medicum quondam felicis recordationis domini Nicolai pape quarti qui fuit primus de ordine minorum.*'

Although the subdeaconate had traditionally been a sacred office, it seems that during the pontificate of Nicholas IV it mainly involved medical duties.[15] The first pontificate to demonstrate the existence of a 'papal doctor' was that of Innocent III (1198–1216).[16] Various famous physicians were employed by popes for their medical services; it is notable that, according to the sources, we can attest more than seventy papal physicians serving at the thirteenth-century court at one time or another.[17] Thus Simon's project regarding the writing of *Clavis* must have played a significant role in his entering and getting the support of the highly medicalized thirteenth-century papal court.

He finished his work after the death of the Pope Nicholas IV and seems to have spent at least two years at the papal curia under Boniface VIII (1296 – 1303).[18] This may be deduced from his reference to Campano of Novara, a famous astrologer, mathematician, and physician, who served the papal court initially under Pope Innocent IV (1243 – 1254), remaining at the curia until his death in September 1296. Simon must have benefited a great deal from the presence of other scholars at the papal court. In referring to Campano he confirms that the latter not only encouraged him in writing the *Clavis* but also provided him with valuable comments.[19] Finally, the success of Simon's time in Rome is further

---

15 On the transformation of the office of the subdiaconate, see Charles Hilken, "Necrological Evidence of the Place and Permanence of the Subdiaconate." In Kathleen G. Cushing and Richard F. Guyg (Eds.), *Ritual, Text, and Law: Studies in Medieval Canon Law and Liturgy Presented to Roger E. Reynolds.* (Aldershot: Ashgate, 2004), 51-66.

16 The 'papal doctor', *medicus papae*, of Innocent III was Master Giovanni Castellomata. On Castellomata's engagement by the papal court see, Agostino Paravicini-Bagliani, *The Pope's Body.* (Chicago; London: University of Chicago Press, 2000), 186-187; and Paravicini-Bagliani, *Medicina e scienze della natura alla corte dei papi nel Duecento.* (Spoleto: Centro italiano di studi sull'alto Medioevo 1991), 217.

17 Cf. Paravicini-Bagliani, *Medicina e scienze della natura...*, 3-51.

18 *Clavis*, preface, § 2: '[...] medicum quondam felicis memorie domini Nicolai pape quarti: qui fuit primus de ordine minorum. [...]' A great many translations of medical works were sponsored in the pontificate of Boniface VII further contributing to the enrichment of medical knowledge; see Paravicini-Bagliani, *The Pope's Body*, 225-234. According to some surviving manuscripts, Simon, with the help of the Jewish-Spanish scholar Abraham of Tortosa (died c. 1330) translated three Arabic treatise into Latin. Two of them are related to simples: a) Abulcasis, *Liber servitoris de preparacione medicinarum simplicium*, and b) Serapion, *Liber aggregratus in medicinis simplicibus*. The third work is an Arabic version of the sixth book of Hippocrates' *Epidemics*. Since, as far as I know, even the necessary philological study has not yet been done, I have not included the aforementioned works in my study. For a general discussion of the translations in connection with Simon's biographical details, see Jacquart, "Arabisants du Moyen Age et de la Renaissance...", 163-164; and Paravicini-Bagliani, *Medicina e scienze della natura...*, 197-198.

19 *Clavis*, preface, § 1: '*Opusculum iam dudum a vobis postulatum quasi quid utile continens cum quanta potui dilligentia qualitercumque ad finem usque perductum ingenio vestro dirigere censui iudicandum* [...].' On Campano of Novara and his medical activity at the papal court, see Paravicini-Bagliani, *The Pope's Body*, 189-190.

attested by his possession of a canonry at Rouen and an ecclesiastical benefice at the cathedral of Padua, which must have been given to him by the Pope in recognition of his services.[20]

Clavis sanationis

Having given an overview of Simon's connection with the thirteenth-century papal court, I shall now return to the *Clavis sanationis*, the *Key of healing*.[21] Simon reports that he spent almost thirty years completing his project, in the course of which he undertook many research trips.[22] His great spirit of enquiry is also attested by his attempts to establish connections with scholars from other countries such as Roger Bacon (c. 1214 – 1294) in order to check rare manuscripts and thus different versions of various terms.[23] The *Clavis* was written after consulting a great number of texts with significant variations in length, style, and credibility.[24] The pharmacological entries consist of a heterogeneous mix of details derived from Greek and Latin sources such as Dioscorides, Cassius Felix (fl. fifth century AD), Alexander of Tralles (c. 525 – 605 AD), or even the twelfth-century Italian translator Stephen of Antioch. Among the Islamic authors,

---

20 The reference to the canonry at Rouen can be found in Simon's preface, *Clavis*, § 2: '*Venerabile viro magistro Simoni Ianuensi domini pape subdiacono et capellano canonico Rothomagensi* [...].' On the ecclesiastical benefice at Padua, see Fritz Schillmann, *Die Formularsammlung des Marinus von Eboli.* (Rom: W. Regenberg 1929), I, nn. 3133 and 3134; and Paravicini-Bagliani, *Medicina e scienze della natura...*, 192, n.39.

21 For a general overview of the work, see Moritz Steinschneider, "Zur Literatur der Synonyma." In Julius Leopold Pagel (Ed.), *Die Chirurgie des Heinrich von Mondeville.* (Berlin: A. Hirschwald, 1892), 590-591; and Hermann Fischer, *Mittelalterliche Pflanzenkunde.* (Hildesheim: G. Olms, 1967), 71-74.

22 *Clavis*, preface, § 4: '[...] *ut per triginta ferme annos quicquid ad id fieri potuit non obmisi* [...].'

23 Roger Bacon records that he had received Simon's requests regarding a Jewish antidotarium and a text of Averroes. Roger Bacon, 'De erroribus medicorum." In Andrew G. Little, Edward T. Withington (Eds.), *Opera hactenus inedita*, IX. (Oxford: Clarendon Press,1928), 172: '[...] *et Symon vidit antidotarium Cosme et Damiani in Ytalia et alia antiqua, et querit antidotarium de Alap quod est in Hebreo, et practicam Aueroys.*'

24 See the entry *Kirtas*, in which Simon refers to his visits to various monasteries in order to research manuscripts, *Clavis*, s.v. *Kirtas*: '[...] *et sic linitas quoddam glutine appellantes pollibant sic que volumina faciebant, et ego vidi Rome in gazofilatiis antiquorum monasteriorum libros et privilegia ex hac materia scripta ex litteris apud nos non intelligibilibus* [...].' On the manuscripts which seem to have been consulted by Simon and survive nowadays, see Paravicini-Bagliani, *Medicina e scienze della natura...*, 193 and 250. For example, he knew both versions of Dioscorides' *De Materia Medica*, including the fifth-century translation and the 11th-c. elaborated version of the text; see Riddle, *Proceedings ...*, 204-9; and Paravicini-Bagliani, *Medicina e scienze della natura...*, 192-193.

we can find Rhazes (865 – 925 AD), Abulcasis (936 – 1013 AD), Avicenna (c. 980 – 1037 AD), and others.[25] There are also less rational medical texts such as the *Kyranides* – a popular Greek collection of magical remedies, which has its origins in the first or second century AD.[26]

Simon's pharmacological awareness and his great concern to provide accurate data is clear in his introductory statement: 'Regarding all simple medicines that are classified into three categories, namely plants, animals, and minerals, it is not enough to rely only on our knowledge of the writings, when we could apportion frequent visits and careful inquiry to support this study, as it is very much related to the diversity among plants.'[27] Observation was not of primary importance in pre-Renaissance medicine and authors usually adopted passages uncritically. However, Simon feels it necessary to cross-check textual evidence with personal observation. A reference to his encounter with a woman from Crete, where he had the chance to check some herbs, is a remarkable illustration of his words.[28]

To provide a convenient starting point for the discussion of certain entries, it is important to mention that of the 770 entries starting with 'A', 581, i.e. almost 75%, contain some pharmacological connotation. The percentage remains roughly the same throughout the entire work. Simon mainly uses two terms to signify a medicament: *farmakon* and *medicamen*. *Farmakon* is a complex medicament, usually made up of various ingredients: a compound drug. He goes even further when he applies the term to a more specific category of drug, classified according to its action: e.g. 'however, we appropriate this name to laxatives'.[29] This is probably due to popular use of various kinds of purgatives

---

25 An overview of his sources is presented in his preface, see *Clavis*, preface, § 4. See also Bertha Gutiérrez Rodilla, "El plumero: la 'Clavis sanationis', de Simón de Cordo (siglo XIII)". *Panacea* 5 (2004): 287-288, who provides a short discussion of the various authors cited by Simon.

26 For example, see *Clavis*, s.v *Strutho cameleos*: '*Strutho cameleos grece strutio avis deformis si avis dici potest apud kiranidam strutho cameleon, arabice vero vocatur naham.*'

27 All translations of Latin are my own. *Clavis*, preface, § 5: '*Triplici existente omnium medicinarum simplicium genere plantarum videlicet animalium et mineralium non satis ad eorum cognitionem solis scripturis innitendum deputaverim quando frequenti visitatione ac diligenti investigatione ad id studium impendatur, quam maxime circa plantarum distantias* [...].'

28 *Clavis* preface, § 4: '[...] *Nec his solum contentus sed ad diversas mundi partes per sedulos viros indagare ab advenis sciscitari non piguit usque adeo quod per montes arduos nemorosas convalles campos ripasque sepe lustrando aliquando comitem me feci cuiusdam anicule cretensis admodum sciole non modo in dignoscendis herbis et nominibus grecis exponendis* [...].'

29 *Clavis*, s.v. *Farmakon*: '*Farmakon medicamentum maxime compositum: nos autem laxativis appropriavimus hoc nomen* [...].'

thought to remove the noxious humors and bring balance to the body according to humoral theory. However, when he refers to drugs, he generally chooses to use the current Latin term *medicamen*, indicating either a healing substance, a remedy, or an antidote.[30]

The majority of the relevant substances described in the *Clavis* as having therapeutic properties can be identified with relative certainty. They are divided into five large groups: a) substances of plant origin, b) substances of animal origin, c) substances of mineral origin, d) *composita*, and e) *preparata*. More than four hundred different species of plants can be identified in the *materia medica*. The inclusion of large numbers of animal products taken from mammals, birds, fish, reptiles, and amphibians, but also various species of insects, is noticeable.[31] Furthermore, although the identification of particular minerals is often uncertain, there is a clear attempt to enumerate Arabic terms for substances of mineral origins, mostly without any explanatory details.[32] The fourth group deals with compound drugs. Details of preparation and dosage are not usually given and many of them have specific names such as *Collirium theodoricon* or *Talasa mellis*. The last group, *preparata*, consists of a large number of substances such as oil, wine, honey, butter, and flour which can either be used alone or as ingredients in a compound drug.

We can also note a considerable variety of pharmaceutical dosage forms. Simon considers it important to give an explanation of each type before he makes further use of it. For example, we see that among the entries beginning with 'T', there are seventeen different kinds of lozenges (*trociscus*). Before he mentions the first lozenge dosage form, he provides a short reference to the word *trociscus*: 'lozenge in Greek is called *trochos*, which is a wheel or something resembling a round [object]. Cassius Felix calls *rotulas* what Greeks call *trociscus* and so on.'[33] Simon usually mentions the Latin equivalent in addition to some morphological characteristics such as shape. There are also cases where we have a quite long description, such as for eye drops. He gives details on both

---

30 For example, see *Clavis*, s.v. *Citron*: '*Citron medicamen ad splenem quod scribitur a Cassius Felix capitulo de splene;*' *Clavis*, s.v. *Echeon*: '*Echeon apud Plinius vocatur medicamen ad visum quod fit ex cinere vipere vive cinerate et melle et succo feniculi;*' and *Clavis* s.v. *Antidotum*: '*Antidotum liber de doctrina greca, antidotos remedium medicamen levamen adiutorium.*'

31 For instance, there are seven different entries dealing with frogs, referring to at least three different species: *Clavis*, s.v. *Batracos, Difdhah, Gecazum, Girinos, Miosos, Vatrachos,* and *Vatrachi kampite.*

32 *Clavis*, s.v. *Hager alcamar*: '*Hager alcamar lapis lune;*' and *Clavis*. s.v. *Hager alsfengi*: '*Hager alsfengi lapis spongie.*'

33 *Clavis*, s.v. *Trociscus*: '*Trociscus dictus a trochos greco quod est rota vel aliquid simile rotundum Cassius Felix rotulas quas greci trociscos vocant et cetera.*'

administration and preparation: 'collirium is an ophthalmic drug of oblong shape which is rubbed on a whetstone [and diluted] with any liquid when it is placed in the eyes and Arabs call it *sief*.'[34] Simon refers to more than fifteen different forms in total including various types of plasters, pills, suppositories, and decoctions.

Since the length of entries varies considerably, my study is based on some characteristic examples of data, which are commonly encountered in the work. These are divided into the following categories:

I. Synonyms
II. Etymological Data
III. Descriptive Data
IV. Healing Uses
V. Empirical Statements[35]

Each group will be examined individually below.

I. Synonyms

One of the most commonly found types of information in the dictionary is a list of synonyms. For example, there are cases of simple disjunction where different names are given in Latin for the same substance such as '*calcitis* and *calciteos* or *calcididos* [...].'[36] But by far the most common examples concern entries with details of synonyms in Greek and Arabic. There are straightforward cases such as '*hager* is the Arabic word for stone' where a direct Latin synonym is provided for an Arabic term.[37] This attests Simon's efforts to include a number of mostly

---

34 *Clavis*, s.v. *Collirium*: '*Collirium est medicina ocularis forma oblonga que fricatur super cotem cum aliquo liquore quando in oculis ponitur et dicitur arabice sief* [...].'

35 The methodology follows the approach used by Stannard in his studies on Byzantine and late medieval pharmacological and botanological lexicography (Jerry Stannard "Byzantine Botanical Lexicography." Episteme 5 (1971): 168-187; "Botanical Data and Late Medieval 'Rezeptliteratur.' In Gundolf Keil et al (Eds.), *Fachprosa-Studien: Beiträge zur mittelalterlichen Wissenschafts- und Geistesgeschichte*. (Berlin: E. Schmidt, 1982), 371-395; "Aspects of Byzantine Materia Medica". *Dumbarton Oaks Papers* 38 (1985): 205-211). One might suggest additional categories corresponding to less common or rare details such as supplementary explanatory anatomical details. For example see *Clavis*, s.v. *Alcula*: '*Alcula vel alcola arabice pustule ulcerose que in ore et lingua fiunt.*' However, this study focuses on details related primarily to pharmacology or connected with the properties and the identification of a pharmacological substance rather than inductive explanations of certain terms mentioned in the entry.

36 *Clavis*, s.v. *Calcitis*: '*Calcitis et calciteos vel calcididos* [...].'

37 *Clavis*, s.v. *Hager*: '*Hager arabice Lapis inde hec.*'

Arabic terms and substances that were not widely known at that period in the West. We can also observe some cross-referencing between entries. In the case of *Agalugim*, we can see Simon referring to its Greek synonym, *xiloaloes*: '[...] *agalosia* is *xiloaloes* [...].'[38] As we will see later, the Greek word is also discussed alone in a separate entry. Thus, Simon provides interconnections between individual entries facilitating his readers' recognition of various names and quick searches.

Furthermore, there are more complicated examples with a long list of synonyms. These entries consist of various versions of the same substance as found in a variety of languages and sources: '*Atriplex* is called in Greek *andrafaxis* and in Dioscorides *crisolacana*, and in Latin that means *aureum olus*. In Arabic it is called *kataf* and *sarmeth*, for which Stephen writes *coatutum* and *sermach*.'[39] Simon gives the common Latin term, which is accompanied by two Greek words, both found in Dioscorides.[40] Then he provides a literal Latin translation of the word, i.e. *aureum olus* (golden vegetable), which is followed by the current Arabic equivalent and the versions that can be found in Stephen of Antioch's *Synonyma*.[41] This entry is also indicative of Simon's compiling methods. He uses a variety of sources just for a single word, comparing different versions. His decision to name the authors of earlier works should not be considered a mere copying technique, but a systematic attempt to provide a kind of brief reference for his readers and enhance the credibility of his words.

II. Etymological Data

Simon sometimes supplies the various synonyms with a short etymological explanation. Connecting the etymology of the name of a substance with its uses had long ago been abandoned. Thus Simon does not relate names to healing

---

38 *Clavis*, s.v. *Agalugim*: '[...] *agalosia est xiloaloes* [...]'.

39 *Clavis*, s.v. *Atriplex*: '*Atriplex grece vocatur andrafaxis apud Dyascoridem et crisolacana, et est dictu aureum olus ut infra, sed arabice kataf et sarmeth dicitur. Stephanus coatutum et sermach.*'

40 Dioscorides, II, 119.

41 Stephen of Antioch or Pisa was an Italian translator of Arabic works, who was active in Antioch in the first part of the twelfth centarury. He is also the author of *Synonyma Stephani*, a trilingual glossary, in Latin, Greek (in Latin characters), and Arabic, of technical terms arranged alphabetically in parallel columns, which remains unedited. For a short description of Stephen's glossary, see MacKinney "Medieval medical dictionaries and glossaries...", 265-266. On Stephen's works and activity, see Charles Burnett "Stephen, the Disciple of Philosophy, and the Exchange of Medical Learning in Antioch". *Crusades* 5 (2006): 113-129.

properties, but specifies various names of the same plant in order to make clear the association of names with particular substances. A good example is the word *Xiloaloes*. As I have shown above, readers can see its synonymous versions without searching for the word itself. If the reader decides to do so, there is a short etymological phrase explaining that it is 'the Greek term for the wood of aloe'. Thus Simon simply gives the literal Latin translation corresponding to the two-part compound, i.e. ξύλον (wood) and ἀλόη (aloe).[42]

An etymology also serves an additional purpose: to indicate the nature and origin of a particular substance. This is clearly shown when he discusses the etymology of the compound drug *Talasa mellis*. He provides an etymologically elaborate comment explaining the first word, that is *talasa*: '[...] the name itself is a compound of Greek *talasa*, which means sea, and honey; for it is sea-water that is used in this preparation [...]'.[43] Thus, Simon is clearly not interested in providing an etymology of a 'philological' nature, but only to facilitate the correct preparation of the drug.

III. Descriptive Data

There are some entries containing descriptive data such as the recognition, origin, and preparation of certain substances for use in their own or as ingredients of compound drugs. The first group of such details deals with botanological identification. For example, Simon compares one plant to another: '*Gariofilata* is a plant similar to *agrimonie* [...]'.[44] For Simon, it is quite usual to supply details in relation to geographical origin and habitat. It normally takes the form of a very general description as in the case of *Costum* ('it is found in many locations') or a more specific geographical location such as in the case of *Cabrusium* ('from the island of Cyprus'), indicating a plant native to Cyprus.[45] Moreover we have cases

---

42 *Clavis*, s.v. *Xiloaloes*: '*Xiloaloes grece lignum aloes*'. See also, Petros Bouras-Vallianatos, '*Xiloaloes*,' with English translation and commentary in *Simon Online*, (www.simonofgenoa. org/index.php5?title=Xiloaloes, 2011): 'The word is in the genitive case following the most common type of case for the ingredients of compound drugs. Greek υ /y/ is phonetically transcribed into the itacist 'ii' and pronounced accordingly. Although an interior elision would normally be expected to occur (with the expulsion of the omikron ο /o/ in ξύλον / *xylon*/ before the alpha α /a/ in ἀλόη /aloe/), Simon's form retains the omicron ο /o/ by analogy with the orthography of other entries beginning with the compound stem /xilo-/, such as *Xilobalsamum* or *Xilocarti*.

43 *Clavis*, s.v. *Talasa mellis*: '[...] docet et est compositum nomen a talasa quod est mare et melle nam aqua maris in ea confectione ingreditur [...].'

44 *Clavis*, s.v. *Gariofilata*: '*Gariofilata est planta similis agrimonie* [...].'

45 *Clavis*, s.v. *Costum*: '[...] invenitur autem in multis locis [...];' and *Clavis*, s.v. *Cabrusium*: '[...] et est dictum cyprense a cypro insula [...].'

of ancient binomials, where the adjective denotes a country or province (e.g. *Vinum creticum* and *Macedonicum oxilatrum*).

By far the longest descriptions are usually connected with morphological features of plants or plant extracts. This may take the form of a short qualifying statement (e.g. 'costum has a bitter root') or a long phrase mostly adopted from Dioscorides (e.g. 'according to Dioscorides the *tragagantum* root is broad and woody, and has short, strong branches that spread over the ground etc.').[46] Sometimes these descriptions may include rather subjective characteristics as in the case of *Ebenus*, where the wood appears 'black' and 'solid', but also 'beautiful'.[47] There are also a limited number of cases that include a long discussion, such as in the case of the *Yris* where Simon uses various comparative criteria such as smell and taste in order to identify three different species, i.e. 'Macedonian', 'Illyrian', and 'Libyan'.[48] As I have shown, recognition of certain plants could clearly have been facilitated by comparing them with various morphological features in plants of the same family or genus. However, it is noteworthy that Simon's dictionary does not constitute a botanological inventory and it does not have the form of Dioscorides' text, which provided such features in every single entry. These kinds of details are encountered only in a certain number of entries and probably occur only when the identification of a particular substance was questionable by the standards of the day.

IV. Healing Uses

An essential part of Simon's information relates to various healing uses. This kind of information is usually very brief and is provided either by an indirect or direct statement. For many entries the relevant chapter of the book from which the data had been taken was indicated, thus: either '*Achates* [...] Alexander in the composition of hydrocollyriums', or '*Anchusa* [...] Paul's chapter on

46 *Clavis*, s.v. *Costum*: '*Costum radix amara* [...];' and *Clavis*, s.v. *Tragagantum*: '*Tragagantum Diascorides radix est lata et lignosa virgas habet breves et fortes et super terram declives in quibus virgis folia sunt plurima et minuta que circa se spinas multas et subcelatas habet que specie albe sunt et fortes radix eius cum maturaverit ferro percussa lachrymum emittit que in sole coagulatur et tragagantum appellatur.* [...]'

47 *Clavis*, s.v. *Ebenus*: '*Ebenus sive ebanus lignum cuius interius nigrum solidum pulchrum* [...].'

48 *Clavis*, s.v. *Yris*: '[...] *pendentes sicande sunt melior est tamen macedonica yris an ylirica et maxime durior et colore ruffo et odore bono. Eligenda est gustu calidior que cum tunditur sternutamenta producit, libica etiam albidior est et gustu amarior* [...].'

dysentery [...]', or 'Berilon [...] in the decoctions for paralysis [...]'.[49] Although no direct statement concerning a particular use is provided, the reader is given the necessary details in order to relate the substance to the treatment of a specific disease. The most common example of entries, which use a direct statement, have the following simple form: either 'Antimonium [...] is an ophthalmic drug [...]' or 'ebenus [...] suitable for eye medicines [...]'.[50] Furthermore, we can find cases with entries that contain therapeutic properties similar to those of another plant. For example, 'Tragagantum [...] its healing virtue is similar to the paremplastic nature of gum [...]' or 'Armech [...] is an Indian medicine similar to cinnamon [...]'.[51] The reader is able to understand and connect the use of a substance with one that is already familiar to them. Thus, Simon's work provides essential information about substances of previously unspecified use. Finally, we may sporadically find various forms of the word 'efficient' either as a noun efficacia or an adjective efficacius in connection with the effectiveness of certain substances.[52]

We can see that the space allowed for the various uses is usually restricted to one little phrase or simply a word. Thus, compared to the usually much longer space allowed for the descriptive data, it may seem weird to modern tastes. However, we have to bear in mind that in ancient and medieval medicine most substances had a healing property and paramount importance was given to the process of distinguishing and administering the most suitable substance.

V. Empirical Statements

And last of all there is another type of information occasionally found and included for reasons similar to those already discussed: empirical statements showing Simon's concern to provide the reader with the most useful details resulting from his considerable research and practical experience. It is striking that among other entries, he feels it necessary to give a short explanation of the

---

49 Clavis, s.v. Achates lapis: 'Achates lapis [...] Alexander in confectione ydrocollirii;' Clavis, s.v. Anchusa: 'Anchusa [...] Paulus capitulo de dissinteria [...];' and Clavis, s.v. Berilon: 'Berilon [...] in decoctione ad paralisim [...].'

50 Clavis, s.v. Antimonium: 'Antimonium [...] est medicina ocularis [...];' and Clavis, s.v. Ebenus: 'Ebenus [...] aptum ocularibus medicis [...].'

51 Clavis, s.v. Tragagantum: 'Tragagantum [...] virtus est ei similis gummi et paremplaustica et cetera [...];' and Clavis, s.v. Armech: 'Armech [...] est medicina inda similis cinamomo [...].'

52 For example, see Clavis, s.v. Acacia: '[...] nos vero tali acacia carentes de fructu prunellarum silvestrium succo expresso et de cocto ad spissitudinem facimus et invenitur in ea efficacia [...].'

Greek word *Empyria*: '*Empyria* is Greek for experience, prudence, the wisdom [coming from] experience'.[53]

The most obvious case is when he uses the first-person singular, in an attempt to increase the plausibility of his words, by providing a personal tone to his statement. A couple of interesting examples, which also illustrate Simon's scholarly approach, are: 'I found it in some book of ancient synonyms in the form *ginda* which is in Latin *iusquiamus*, but I do not know whether they are the same' or 'I have never seen or heard of anyone who has seen it'.[54] In a similar vein, when he refers to the use of swallow's stones, which were usually employed as an amulet against various diseases, he reports that he had only found white stones in contrast to the sources which mention a black and a red stone.[55] Although he must have encountered a great number of the substances he mentions in the course of his career, he sometimes supplements an entry with a direct statement regarding the medicinal activity of particular substances. For example, referring to certain species of the *Yris*, he states that '[...] as for medicinal strength it is only in the second division [...]'.[56] Thus, it is important to mention that Simon's statements were not only authenticated by the juxtaposition of information from textual sources, oral sources, and actual observation, but also by the fact that he was a practicing physician.

Conclusions

The *Clavis sanationis* constitutes an ambitious project, which clearly fulfilled a contemporary need. It is not a *vade mecum* with selected and effective recipes and it cannot replace the texts of its cited authors. The *Clavis* has the primary function of providing a quick-reference guide to well-chosen details for substances otherwise scattered among a great number of sources. We can only imagine the difficulty of collecting and collating so many different manuscripts and recording findings without the use of modern technology. Moreover, the constant refining of the data provided thanks to his personal wealth of experience, making the work unique for its time. The rich afterlife of Simon's work, attested

---

53 *Clavis*, s.v. *Empyria*: '*Empyria grece experientia prudentia exercitatio paritia prudentia.*'
54 *Clavis*, s.v. *Ginga*: '*Ginga* [...] *invenio in antiquis synonimis ginda quod est iusquiamum, an sit idem nescio;*' and *Clavis*, s.v. *Costum*: '*Costum* [...] *invenitur autem in multis locis costum dulce scriptum in confectionibus, sed nec vidi nec audivi ab aliquo vidisse.*'
55 *Clavis*, s.v. *Lapis Chelidoneus*: '*Lapis chelidoneus invenitur in ventribus yrundinum: cuius genera sunt duo, niger et ruffus qui colliguntur captis pulis yrundinum ex nido et fixis eorum ventribus invenitur et cetera, ego vero inveni cum his et albos* [...].'
56 *Clavis*, s.v. *Yris*: '[...] *hec in virtute ponitur in secundo loco* [...].'

by numerous references in later pharmacopoeias of the succeeding centuries, confirms its widespread use.[57] Finally, the fact that it has preserved a huge number of names and their relationship with known substances could prove vitally important in the future study of as yet unpublished early Renaissance or late Byzantine pharmacological works.

---

[57] An abridged version of Simon's *Clavis* appeared as early as the fourteenth century; see Collins, *Medieval Herbals.*, 269-70, who discusses one of the earliest surviving manuscripts, *Parisinus Latinus* 6823, of this version. Around the middle of the 15th c., Saladin of Ascoli, physician to the prince of Taranto, included *Clavis* among six texts, which he suggested should be used by contemporary apothecaries; see Teresa Huguet-Termes, "Islamic Pharmacology and Pharmacy in the Latin West: An Approach to Early Pharmacopoeias". *European Review* 16 (2008): 229-239. One more notable example can be found in the Florentine *Nuovo Receptario*, the oldest 'pharmacopoeia', published in 1498, which considers Simon's Clavis a prerequisite for the establishment of a new apothecary; see Anna Maria Carmona i Cornet, *Nuovo Receptario Composto dal Famossisimo Chollegio degli Eximii Doctori della Arte et Medicina della Inclita Cipta di Firenze.* (Barcelona: Institut Mèdico-Farmacèutic de Catalunya, 1992) 6r.

Bibliography

d'Alverny, Marie-Thérèse. "Translations and Translators." In Robert L. Benson and Giles Constable (Eds.), *Renaissance and Renewal in the Twelfth Century.* 421-462. Cambridge: Harvard University Press, 1982.

Bacon, Roger. "De erroribus medicorum." In Andrew. G. Little and Edward. Withington (Eds.), *Opera hactenus inedita*, IX. 150-179. Oxford: Clarendon Press, 1928.

Burnett, Charles. "Stephen, the Disciple of Philosophy, and the Exchange of Medical Learning in Antioch." *Crusades* 5 (2006): 113-129.

Carmona i Cornet, Anna Maria. *Nuovo Receptario Composto dal Famossisimo Chollegio degli Eximii Doctori della Arte et Medicina della Inclita Cipta di Firenze.* Barcelona: Institut Mèdico-Farmacèutic de Catalunya, 1992.

Collins, Minta. *Medieval Herbals.* London: British Library and University of Toronto, 2000.

Dioscorides. *De Materia medica*, edited by Max Wellmann. Berlin: Weidmann, 1907.

Fischer, Hermann. *Mittelalterliche Pflanzenkunde.* Hildesheim: G. Olms, 1967.

Fortuna, Stefania. "Pietro d'Abano e le traduzioni Latine di Galeno." *Medicina nei Secoli* 20 (2008): 447-463.

García González, Alejandro. *Alphita.* Firenze: SISMEL edizioni del Galluzzo, 2008.

Goltz, Dietlinde. *Mittelalterliche Pharmazie und Medizin. Dargestellt an Geschichte und Inhalt des Antidotarium Nicolai.* Stuttgart: Wissenschaftliche Verlagsgesellschaft, 1976.

Gutiérrez Rodilla, Bertha. "El plumero: la 'Clavis sanationis', de Simón de Cordo (siglo XIII)." *Panacea* 5 (2004): 287-288.

Hein, Wolfgang-Hagen and Kurt Sappert. *Die Medizinalordnung Friedrichs: Eine pharmaziehistorische Studie.* Eutin: Internationale Gesellschaft für Geschichte der Pharmazie, 1957.

Hilken, Charles. "Necrological Evidence of the Place and Permanence of the Subdiaconate." In Kathleen G. Cushing and Richard F. Guyg (Eds.), *Ritual, Text, and Law: Studies in Medieval Canon Law and Liturgy Presented to Roger E. Reynolds.* 51-66. Aldershot: Ashgate, 2004.

Huguet-Termes, Teresa. "Islamic Pharmacology and Pharmacy in the Latin West: An Approach to Early Pharmacopoeias." *European Review* 16 (2008): 229-239.

Jacquart, Danielle. "Arabisants du Moyen Age et de la Renaissance: Jérôme Ramusio († 1486) correcteur de Gérard de Crémone († 1187)." *Bibliothèque de l'École des Chartes* 147 (1989): 399-415.

Jacquart, Danielle and Françoise Micheau. *La médecine arabe et l'Occident médiéval.* Paris: Maissonneuve et Larose, 1990.

Keil, Gundolf. "Zur Datierung des Antidotarium Nicolai." *Sudhoffs Archiv* 62 (1978): 190-6.

MacKinney, Loren C. "Medieval medical dictionaries and glossaries." In Lea James Cate and Eugene Anderson (Eds.), *Medieval historiographical essay: in honor of James Westfall Thompson.* 240-268. Chicago: The University of Chicago Press, 1938.

Marangon, Paolo, "Per una revisione dell'interpretazione di Pietro d'Abano." In Paolo Marangon (Ed.), *Il pensiero ereticale nella Marca Trevigiana e a Venezia dal 1200 al 1350.* 66-104. Abano Terme, Padova: Francisci, 1984.

Paravicini-Bagliani, Agostino. *Medicina e scienze della natura alla corte dei papi nel Duecento.* Spoleto: Centro italiano di studi sull'alto Medioevo, 1991.

— *The Pope's Body.* Chicago: University of Chicago Press, 2000.

Riddle, John M. "The Latin Alphabetical Dioscorides Manuscript Group." *Proceedings of the XIIIth International Congress for the History of Science, Acts Section* IV (1974): 204-209.

Schillmann, Fritz. *Die Formularsammlung des Marinus von Eboli. Rom*: W. Regenberg, 1929.

Stannard, Jerry. "Byzantine Botanical Lexicography". *Episteme* 5 (1971): 168-187.

— Botanical Data and Late Medieval 'Rezeptliteratur'. In Gundolf Keil et al (Eds.), Fachprosa-Studien: *Beiträge zur mittelalterlichen Wissenschafts- und Geistesgeschichte.* 371-395. Berlin: E. Schmidt, 1982.

— "Aspects of Byzantine *Materia Medica.*" *Dumbarton Oaks Papers* 38 (1985): 205-211.

Steinschneider, Moritz. "Zur Literatur der Synonyma." In Julius Leopold Pagel (Ed.), *Die Chirurgie des Heinrich von Mondeville.* 582- 595. Berlin: A. Hirschwald, 1892.

Strohmaier, Gotthard. "Constantine's pseudo-Classical terminology and its survival." In Charles Burnett and Danielle Jacquart (Eds.), *Constantine the African and ʾAlī Ibn al-ʾAbbās al-Maǧdūsī.* 90-98. Leiden: Brill, 1994.

Thorndike, Lynn. "Translations of Works of Galen from the Greek by Peter of Abano." *Isis* 33 (1942): 649-653.

Siam Bhayro (University of Exeter)

Simon of Genoa as an Arabist[1]

Introduction

At first glance, the Latin transcriptions of Arabic medical terminology in Simon of Genoa's *Clavis* can appear eccentric and unpredictable, differing markedly from what is attested in Classical Arabic. After a brief introduction to the phenomenon we call 'Middle Arabic'[2], we shall discuss five features of MA that commonly occur in Simon's Latin transcriptions. We shall show that Simon's transcriptions conform to MA and are, therefore, entirely predictable. We shall then move from a linguistic to an historical analysis, by considering Simon's use of sources, both written and oral, and try to discern the extent of his knowledge of Arabic.

Middle Arabic

The term MA should not be understood in the sense of Middle Aramaic or Middle English – it does not refer to a phase, but rather a register, of the language. The study of the phenomenon we call MA has been plagued by misunderstandings and arguments over definitions, partly because the pioneer of this field was forced to change his initial use of the term following reviews of his early publications.[3] While

---

1 I would like to thank Dr. Barbara Zipser (Royal Holloway University of London), who suggested that I write about this topic and provided much assistance, both by correspondence and through her *Simon Online* web page (simonofgenoa.org) from which the examples given below are drawn. I would also like to thank *Simon Online* author Wilf Gunther, who has contributed greatly to the project, especially in relation to the Arabic terminology. The entries quoted in this article were edited by Gunther, with the exception of *C littera* and *Harsas* (Zipser) and *Gemus* (me). The collation is based on witnesses ABC (prints) and ef (manuscripts), as referenced on *Simon Online*. For the sake of clarity, trivial variants and readings that are clearly errors transmitted in only one source will not be mentioned. Abbreviations for lexica (followed by volume/page number): D = Reinhart Dozy, *Supplément aux Dictionnaires Arabes* (2 vols; Leiden: Brill, 1881); L = Edward William Lane, *An Arabic-English Lexicon* (Parts 1-8 and Supplement; London: Williams and Norgate, 1863-1893).

2 Hereafter MA. Other abbreviations for languages: A = Arabic, CA = Classical Arabic, H = Hebrew, J-A = Judaeo-Arabic, N-A/NA = Neo-Arabic.

3 See the discussion in the 'Addenda and Corrigenda' in Joshua Blau, *The Emergence and Linguistic Background of Judaeo-Arabic: A Study of the Origins of Neo-Arabic and Middle Arabic.* (third revised edition; Jerusalem: Ben-Zvi Institute, 1999), 216-218.

the dust has largely settled, some arguments persist.[4] For our present purposes,[5] however, it is expedient to use the term MA, as defined by Joshua Blau:

> Middle Arabic is the language of medieval A texts in which classical, post-classical, and often also N-A and pseudo-correct elements alternate quite freely.[6]

Again, the circumstances that led to the appearance of a literary register of Arabic, essentially a medieval *koine*, are much debated. Blau's description seems to be the most apposite:

> As a rule, the writers wanted to write in the language of prestige, viz. in Classical Arabic, yet, because of their inability to master its complex grammar, elements of their spoken language, viz. Neo-Arabic, penetrated their writings. Yet in the course of time, a certain mixture of Classical and Neo-Arabic elements came to be thought of as a literary language in its own rights, employed even by authors who were well able to write in a 'more Classical' language.[7]

Thus in the thirteenth century, for example, the Islamic medical historian Ibn Abī Uṣaybiʿah wrote his ʿUyūn al-anbāʾ fī ṭabaqāt al-aṭibbāʾ 'Sources of Information about the Classes of Physicians' in MA.[8]

In addition to elements of both the Classical and spoken language, certain features, defined as 'pseudo-corrections', also manifest. These include hypercorrections, half-corrections and malapropisms, and often represent the misapplication of Classical forms.[9]

---

4 For a recent assessment, see Johannes den Heijer, "Introduction: Middle and Mixed Arabic, a New Trend in Arabic Studies," in L. Zack and A. Schippers (Eds), *Middle Arabic and Mixed Arabic: Diachrony and Synchrony.* (Leiden: Brill, 2012), 1–25.

5 This paper is written with the non-specialist in mind. It is, therefore, not so concerned with the intricacies of the debate about Middle Arabic, but more with assisting the non-Arabist in appreciating how, by following a series of clearly defined steps, one can move from the form given in the Classical Arabic lexica to the form attested in Simon's *Clavis*.

6 See Joshua Blau, *A Handbook of Early Middle Arabic* (Jerusalem: The Max Schloessinger Memorial Foundation, 2002), 14. Compare, however, Blau's comments elsewhere: 'I would even propose to discard, when dealing with Middle Arabic, the terms Classical Arabic and Postclassical Arabic, and use in their stead the term Standard Arabic, comprising both of them, since they constituted for these authors a uniform entity. So the final definition for Middle Arabic I am proposing is that it is the language of texts in which Standard Arabic, Neo-Arabic and pseudo-correct elements alternate in ever varying degrees' – see Blau, *Emergence*, 218.

7 Joshua Blau, "The State of Research in the Field of the Linguistic Study of Middle Arabic," *Arabica* 28 (1981): 187-203, 188. Readers may also wish to consult Kees Versteegh, *The Arabic Language* (Edinburgh: Edinburgh University Press, 1997), 114-129.

8 Blau, 'The State of Research', 191.

9 Blau, 'The State of Research', 189.

For two not unrelated reasons, the best sources for the study of MA are usually those produced by non-Muslim writers. First, non-Muslim writers were less likely to have an ideological devotion to the concept of the ʿarabiyya. Thus, Blau states that, 'the study of early MA has to rely to a considerable degree on the literature of the religious minorities of the Muslim empire'.[10] Second, many of the features of MA are not always visible when Arabic script is being used, but are often only noticeable when the language is phonetically transcribed in another script such as Hebrew, Greek, Coptic, or, as discussed below, Latin.[11]

Features of Middle Arabic Present in Simon of Genoa's Transcriptions

Simon's Latin transcriptions of Arabic medical terminology consistently display MA features. In this section, we limit ourselves to the five features that we consider to be the most important, that is those that account for the vast majority of deviations from the known CA form.[12]

(1) Elision of short final vowels, resulting in the absence of case markers

This is perhaps the most prominent feature of MA,[13] yet it remains obscured in most texts and is only noticeable in phonetic transcription. Thus Blau notes that, 'Although the disappearance of the case endings in the sg. and broken pl. is not exhibited in unvocalized script, it is reflected in Greek transcriptions and J-A texts in phonetic H transcription {as well as in the late Coptic transliteration and late vocalized J-A documents} in H characters}'.[14] As the following two examples demonstrate, it is also very clearly attested in Simon's Latin transcriptions:

---

10 Blau, *Handbook*, 19.

11 Indeed, even with Judaeo-Arabic, there are two types of transcription, one orthographic and the other phonetic, with only the latter revealing the MA elements – see Blau, *Handbook*, 22. For an example of an Arabic text in Greek transcription, see Joshua Blau, *A Grammar of Christian Arabic based mainly on South Palestinian Texts from the First Millennium* (3 vols; Louvain: CSCO, 1966), vol. I, 31. For an example in Coptic transcription, see Joshua Blau, "Some Observations on a Middle Arabic Egyptian Text in Coptic Characters." *Jerusalem Studies in Arabic and Islam* 1 (1979), 215-262. See below for examples in Latin transcription.

12 For each example, we give the quotation from the *Clavis* and an explanatory translation. We also give the CA form in both Arabic script and Latin transliteration, as an aid to comparison, with a reference to either Dozy's or Lane's lexicon.

13 And of Arabic in general, except for CA, even from as early as the first Islamic century – see Simon Hopkins, *Studies in the Grammar of Early Arabic based upon Papyri Datable to before A.H. 300/A.D. 912* (Oxford: Oxford University Press, 1984), 155, especially footnote 1 of §161.

14 Blau, *Handbook*, 44.

(a)   *Dimad arabice cataplasma.*
   Dimad is the Arabic word for Latin *cataplasma* ('poultice, plaster').

CA   ضِمَادٌ   ḍimādun (L 1802)

(b)   *Ramad ara. cinis.*
   Ramad is the Arabic word for Latin *cinis* ('ashes').

CA   رَمَادٌ   ramādun (L 1154)

(2)   imāla

This is the term used to describe the vowel shift *a > e/ə/i* and *ā > ē/ī*, except where the vowel occurs in direct contact with, and in the same syllable as, an emphatic (*ṣ, ṭ, ẓ,* or *ḍ*), uvular (*ḵ, ḡ,* or q), pharyngal (ʻ or *ḥ*), or trill (r).[15] As with the previous feature, Blau notes that, 'as a rule the unvocalized MA texts do not reflect this feature... It is only in Violet's Greek transcription... and in J-A texts in phonetic H transcription which often mark short vowels by vowel letters... that it can be clearly attested {and the same applies to late vocalized J-A texts... as well as to late Coptic transcription...}'.[16] As the following examples demonstrate, Simon's Latin transcriptions are valuable in that they clearly show the rules being followed consistently, even in respect to the exceptions. For the non-exceptional cases, consider examples **(c)** and **(d)** below, which also show the elision of short final vowels in keeping with the first feature described above:

(c)   *Belesem ara. balsamum.*
   Belesem is the Arabic word for Latin *balsamum* ('balsam').[17]

CA   بَلَسَانٌ   *balasānun* (L 248)

---

15 There are exceptions for the latter two categories. For the rules in detail, see Hopkins, *Studies*, 4-5, and 8-9.

16 Blau, *Handbook*, 29. For more details regarding the occurrence of *imāla* in J-A and Muslim MA, see Blau, *Emergence*, 73 and 125 respectively. For Christian MA, see Blau, *Grammar*, vol. I, 64-65. For a very detailed discussion of the rules in relation to the text in Coptic script, see Blau, "Some Observations," 222-227.

17 The lemma is not transmitted unanimously. One group of witnesses reads *Belesem*, while the other reads *Belesen*, which could be said to better resemble the Arabic form. Final *–n* and *–m* could easily be confused in the process of copying, however, as both could be written by a line above the final e. Since we do not know whether Simon used a written or oral source for this lemma, we are not able to determine which reading is original.

(d) *Arabes autem habent .d. ut nos quod del vocant nichilominus habent aliud velud aspiratum quod dhel vocant per quod dheheb quod est aurum scribunt.*

The Arabs have 'd' like us, which they call *del*. Notwithstanding they have another sound, aspirated as it were, which they call *dhel* and with which they write the word *dheheb*, which is in Latin *aurum* ('gold').

CA   ذَالْ   *ḏālun* (L 947)

      ذَهَبْ   *ḏahabun* (L 983)

For exceptions relating to the emphatics (*ṣ*, *ṭ*, *ẓ*, and *ḍ*), consider the following four examples.

(e) For *ṣ*:

Kasab arabice canna arundo.

Kasab is the Arabic word for Latin *canna* or *arundo* ('reed, cane').

CA   قَصَبْ   *qaṣabun* (L 2529)

(f) For *ṭ*:

Kataf arabice yrundo.

Kataf is the Arabic word for Latin *yrundo* ('swallow').

CA   خُطّافْ   *ḵuṭṭāfun* (L 766)

As well as the elision of the short final vowel, example **(f)** also shows regressive vowel assimilation (see the fifth feature discussed below), i.e. *ḵuṭṭāfun* > *ḵuṭṭāf* > *ḵaṭṭāf*, realised as *kataf*, thus disguising both the emphatic and doubled nature of the middle consonant.

(g) For *ẓ*:

Handal arabice colloquintida, Ste. hansalum scripsit.

Handal is the Arabic word for Latin *colloquintida* ('colocynth'). Stephanus writes *hansalum*.[18]

CA   خَنْظَلْ   *ḥanẓalun* (L 657)

---

[18] The lemma is not transmitted unanimously. While *Handal* is the majority reading, there is also *Handel* and *Handhel*, which are representing forms with either d or ḍ, respectively, instead of the emphatic *ẓ*, hence the presence of *imāla* in their second syllables.

(h)   For *ḍ*:
Dahan arabice damula.
Dahan is the Arabic word for Latin *damula* ('little goat-like animal').[19]

CA   ضَأْن   *ḍaʿnun* (L 1760)

Example **(h)** also shows a common pseudo-correction that often follows the elision of the short final vowel, namely **CvCC > CvCvC**, with progressive vowel assimilation, i.e. *ḍaʿnun > ḍaʿn > ḍaʿan*, realised as *dahan*.

For exceptions relating to the uvulars (*ḵ*, *ḡ* and *q*), consider the following three examples:

(i)   For *ḵ*:
Kardel arabice sinapis.
Kardel is the Arabic word for Latin *sinapis* ('mustard').

CA   خَرْدَل   *ḵardalun* (L 721)

In example **(i),** both the norm and an exception are being observed, with *imāla* present in the second syllable but not in the first.

(j)   For *ḡ*:
Gar arabice laurus.
Gar is the Arabic word for Latin *laurus* ('laurel tree, bay').

CA   غَاز   *ḡārun* (L 2307-2308)

(k)   For *q*:
Kalb arabice cor.
Kalb is the Arabic word for Latin *cor* ('heart').

CA   قَلْب   *qalbun* (L 2553)

Contrary to example **(h)** above, **(k)** does not show the pseudo-correction **CvCC > CvCvC** following the elision of the short final vowel.

---

[19] There are a number of variants, including *Dhan dan* and *Dham vel dhanadan*, which could suggest that one of the sources was annotated, subsequently causing confusion.

The pharyngals (ʿ and ḥ) sometimes observe the exception, for example:

(l)   For ʿ:
Hambar ara. ambra.
Hambar is the Arabic word for Latin *ambra* ('ambergris').[20]

CA   عَنْبَرٌ   ʿanbarun (L 2168)

For ḥ, see example **(g)** above. The trill *r* will also observe the exception more often than not – see example **(b)** above, which also has progressive vowel assimilation.

(3)   Reduction of final doubled consonant

Another feature of MA readily noticeable in Simon's Latin transcriptions is the shortening of a doubled consonant in final position,[21] which has been left vulnerable following the elision of the short final vowel – see examples **(m)**, which observes *imāla*, and **(n)**, which does not due to the presence of ḵ:

(m)   *Sceb ara. alumen.*
Sceb is the Arabic word for Latin *alumen* ('alum').

CA   شَبٌّ   šabbun (L 1493)

(n)   *Khas arabice lactuca.*
Khas is the Arabic word for Latin *lactuca* ('lettuce').

CA   خَسٌّ   ḵassun (L 736)

(4)   Loss of *tāʾ marbūṭa*

The phenomenon of *tāʾ marbūṭa* occurs in feminine nouns. In the nominative singular, for example, it occurs in the termination –*atun* that results from the restitution of the historic feminine marker *t* to enable the use of the following

---

20 The manuscripts transmit both *Hambar* and *Hambair*. Note also the use of h for Arabic ʿ, which helps us understand example (o) below.
21 Blau, *Handbook*, 31.

case vowel *u*.[22] Like the shortening of a final doubled consonant, the loss of *tā᾿ marbūṭa* is another consequence of the elision of the short final vowel, i.e. the case vowel *u*, which leaves the artificially restored *t* vulnerable, thus *-atun* > *-at* > *-a(h)*, which, depending on the preceding consonant, may change to *-e(h)* on account of *imāla*. The use of *h* would reflect an orthographic rather than phonetic transcription.[23] Simon's approach to transcription appears to be purely phonetic, however, so his forms simply display either *-a* or *-e*:

(o)   With *-a*:
Karaha arabice cucurbita.
Karaha is the Arabic word for Latin *cucurbita* ('gourd').

CA   قَرْعَةٌ   *qarʿatun* (D II.340)

In example **(o)**, the process by which *qarʿatun* becomes *karaha* involves several stages, thus: *qarʿatun* > *qarʿat* (elision of short final vowel) > *qarʿa* (loss of *tā᾿ marbūṭa*) > *qaraʿa* (pseudo-correction, with progressive vowel assimilation), realised as *karaha*, with *k* for *q* and *h* for *ʿ* as already observed in examples **(k)** and **(l)** above. One point of interest here is that the final *-ha* has not been realised as *-he*, on account of the underlying *ʿ*, thus showing much accuracy in the vocalic elements of the phonetic transcription.

(p)   With *-e*:
Cerfe arabice cortex arborum, melius per .k. scribitur.
Cerfe is the Arabic word for Latin *cortex arborum* ('bark of trees'); it is better written with 'k'.

CA   قِرْفَةٌ   *qirfatun* (D II.342)

As with the previous example, **(p)** exhibits several stages: *qirfatun* > *qirfat* (elision of short final vowel) > *qirfa* (loss of *tā᾿ marbūṭa*) > *qirfe* (imāla) > *qerfe* (regressive vowel assimilation), realized as *cerfe*, with *c* for *q* (although Simon prefers *k* – this is discussed further below).

---

22 See, for example, William Wright, *A Grammar of the Arabic Language*, translated from the German of Caspari and edited with numerous additions and corrections (third edition revised by W. Robertson Smith and M. J. de Goeje; 2 vols; Cambridge: Cambridge University Press, 1951), vol. I, 7 (end of §2 and footnote) and 184 (end of §294).
23 For Blau's discussion of this feature of MA, in relation to the text in Coptic transcription, see Blau, "Some Observations," 246.

(5)   Vowel assimilation

Blau notes that: ']-A texts spelt in phonetic transcription reflect cases of assimilation of vowels, both regressive and progressive, not recognisable in texts written in standard orthography'. We have already seen how Simon's Latin transcriptions of Arabic medical terminology are phonetic, rather than orthographic, and are very accurate. It is not surprising, therefore, that both types of vowel assimilation are readily noticeable. For regressive vowel assimilation, see examples **(f)** and **(p)** above; for progressive vowel assimilation, see **(h)** above and also consider the following example:

(q)   *Scahar capillus sed sahar melius et xahar ordeum.*
         Scahar is the Arabic for Latin *capillus* ('hair'), but it is better to write *sahar* and *xahar* meaning Latin *ordeum* ('barley').

CA   شَعِيرٌ   *šaʿīrun* (L 1561)

Thus *šaʿīrun* > *šaʿīr* > *šaʿar*, realised as *scahar*.
From the preceding analysis of five MA features, it is clear, therefore, that Simon's Latin transcriptions are far from random – they are an accurate phonetic representation of MA forms and, as such, are very predictable. Indeed, they are an extremely valuable witness to MA and add to the small corpus of phonetic MA texts hitherto recognised.

Simon's Use of Multiple Arabic Sources and Latin Intermediaries

In addition to their linguistic value, Simon's Latin transcriptions are also of historical interest on account of what they reveal about his knowledge of Arabic and the methods he employed in compiling the *Clavis*.
    Simon names a number of Arabic authorities in his *Clavis*,[24] including Albenmesue,[25] Rasis,[26] Aliabas (Haly Abbas),[27] Abulcasis,[28]

---

24 See the Preface §4 (print A, page 2 f.).
25 I.e. **Abū Zakarīyāʾ Yūḥannā ibn Māsawaih**, who flourished between the late eighth and mid-ninth centuries in Iraq; see Manfred Ullmann, *Die Medizin im Islam* (Leiden: Brill, 1970), 112-115.
26 I.e. **Abū Bakr Muḥammad ibn Zakarīyāʾ ar-Rāzī**, who flourished between the late ninth and early tenth centuries in Iran; see Ullmann, *Die Medizin*, 128-136.
27 I.e. ʿAlī ibn al-ʿAbbās al-Majūsī, who flourished in the late tenth century in Iran; see Ullmann, *Die Medizin*, 140-146.
28 I.e. Abū l-Qāsim Ḳalaf ibn al-ʿAbbās az-Zahrāwī, who flourished between the late tenth and early eleventh centuries in Spain; see Ullmann, *Die Medizin*, 149-151.

Avicenna,[29] and Averroes.[30] He also mentions an Almansor and an Isaac, but these names are too common to permit any identification with certainty.[31] Crucially, Simon also refers to two scholars who translated from Arabic into Latin: Constantinus Africanus, who translated **ar-Rāzī** and **al-Majūsī**,[32] and Stephen of Antioch, who also translated **al-Majūsī**.[33]

Therefore, as one reads through Simon's discussions one notices that, while he refers to multiple Arabic authorities, he is often accessing them only through pre-existing Latin translations. The following two examples illustrate this nicely:

(r) *Cerfe arabice cortex arborum, melius per .k. scribitur.*
Cerfe is the Arabic word for Latin *cortex arborum* ('bark of trees'); it is better written with 'k'.

Kerfe arabice cortex arboris apud Avi. per .c. scribitur sed melius per .k. dicitur etiam kiserech. Avi. duo facit ca. unum de kerfe aromatico aliud de kerfe cinamomi.
Kerfe is the Arabic word for Latin *cortex arboris* ('tree bark'). In Avicenna it is spelled with 'c', but it is better with 'k'. It is also called *kiserech*. Avicenna has two chapters, one on aromatic *kerfe*, the other on cinnamon *kerfe*.

CA   قِرْفَةٌ   *qirfatun* (D II.342)

We can see in example **(r)** that at least two pre-existing sources are being used; each possessing its own preferred Latin spelling. Moreover, when Simon states 'in Avicenna it is spelled with…', he is clearly referring to a Latin translation of **Ibn Sīnā**, not an Arabic copy. If he was using Arabic sources, such a discussion would not even be necessary – the problem only arises because two different Latin sources, each with its own transliteration system, are being employed. Indeed, one wonders whether anyone competent with Arabic would even think to make such a statement – after all, it is certain that **Ibn Sīnā** did not use a 'c'.

---

29 I.e. Abū ʿAlī al-Ḥusain ibn ʿAbd Allāh ibn Sīnā who flourished in the early eleventh century in Iran; see Ullmann, *Die Medizin*, 152-156.

30 I.e. Abū l-Walīd Muḥammad ibn Aḥmad ibn Muḥammad ibn Rušd, who flourished in the late twelfth century in Spain and Morocco; see Ullmann, *Die Medizin*, 166-167.

31 It is possible that Isaac refers to Isaac Judaeus, i.e. Abū Yaʿqūb Isḥāq ibn Sulaymān al-Isrāʾīlī who flourished in the early tenth century in Tunisia; see Ullmann, *Die Medizin*, 137-138.

32 See, for example, Peter E. Pormann and Emilie Savage-Smith, *Medieval Islamic Medicine* (Edinburgh: Edinburgh University Press, 2007), 164. *Constantine also translated Isaac Judaeus*; see Ullmann, *Die Medizin*, 137.

33 See, for example, Pormann and Savage-Smith, *Medieval Islamic Medicine*, 168.

(s) *Scebet ara. anetum.*
Scebet is the Arabic word for Latin *anetum* ('dill, anise').

Sebetum scripsit Ste. pro xebet quod est anetum.
Stephen writes *sebetum* for the Arabic word *xebet*, which in Latin means *anetum* ('dill, anise').

Xebet ara. anetum.
Xebet is the Arabic word for Latin *anetum* ('dill, anise').

CA   شِبْثٌ   *šibṯun* (L 1495)

Again, in example **(s)**, at least three different sources are being used. Furthermore, it is clear that Simon is operating at least one stage removed from the written Arabic sources, relying on a combination of pre-existing Latin sources.

Simon's Knowledge of Arabic

This raises the question of Simon's own knowledge of Arabic – if he is dependent on Latin translations of Arabic sources, can we even refer to Simon as an Arabist?
  There is no evidence in the *Clavis* of a direct knowledge of Arabic on Simon's part. This is not unexpected, however, given the nature of the source. After all, it is very difficult to envisage precisely what would constitute evidence of direct knowledge of Arabic in the *Clavis*. On the other hand, as we have already seen, there is plenty of evidence of the use of a Latin intermediary. Furthermore, there is the occasional suggestion of an ignorance of Arabic on Simon's part, as demonstrated in **(r)** above and in the following example:

(t)   *C littera greci omnino carent et eius sono: latini vero ipsa in grecis dictionibus usi sunt ubi greci .k. vel .X. que chi apud eos sonat scribunt, sed arabes .c. litteram eo sono quo nos proferimus: et ipsi proferunt aliquando maxime occidentales, orientales vero eidem .t. littere sonum attribuunt semper unde orientales dicunt catin quod occidentales cacin vocant et est annulus.*
  The Greeks lack the letter 'c' and its sound: the Latins on the other hand use it in Greek words where the Greeks write 'k' or 'χ', which is pronounced *chi* by them; the Arabs pronounce the letter 'c' as we do. And it is the Westerners who pronounce it most, the Easterners on the other hand give it the same sound as 't'. The Easterners always say *catin* for what the Westerners call *cacin*, and this means 'signet ring'.

CA   خَاتِمٌ   *ḫātimun* (D I.351-352)

In example **(t)**, Simon appears to be suggesting that the noun *ḵātim* 'seal, signet ring'[34] is realised in two different ways: *catin* in the east and *cacin* in the west. This is most unlikely.[35] Indeed, the two distinct forms probably arise from the common confusion between the letters *c* and *t* in Latin manuscripts. Moreover, Simon appears to be giving priority to the form *cacin*, thus showing a total ignorance of the underlying Arabic form.

In addition to showing an ignorance of Arabic, Simon also displays remoteness from the oriental sources. For example:

(u) *Mumia invenitur in sepulchris mortuorum antiquorum et constat ex substantia ipsorum cadaverum et mixtura condimentorum quibus condiebantur sive mirra et aloe sive quibuscumque aliis nobis ignotis.*
Mumia is what is found in the tombs of the dead of antiquity and consists of a substance made of those cadavers with a mixture of spices with which they were embalmed or myrrh or aloe or with whatever other chemicals unknown to us.

CA   مُومِيَا   *mūmiyā* (D II.633)

Contrary to Simon's discussion of the term, *mūmiyā* refers to a type of asphalt or bitumen originating in India, Iran, and Iraq. It is probably an Iranian word that was loaned into both Syriac and Arabic,[36] which could explain why the Iranian scholars **ar-Rāzī** and **ibn Sīnā** were in no doubt as to its true nature.[37] It is clear, therefore, that Simon presents a folk tradition rather than a scientific description.

---

34 Our discussion of this example is slightly hampered by the uncertainty in the modern Arabic lexica regarding this word. Having given the initial gloss as 'anus', Dozy then discusses a reference in the *1001 Nights*, which refers to how the mouth of a beautiful young maiden resembles the *ḵātim* of Solomon, a context for which the gloss 'anus' would not be wholly appropriate. The concept of the signet-ring or seal of Solomon is well known in Jewish Aramaic, possessing associations with wisdom and magical powers. For example, the phrase המלשיד אמתח occurs in an Aramaic magic bowl – see Joseph Naveh and Shaul Shaked, *Magic Spells and Formulae: Aramaic Incantations of Late Antiquity* (Jerusalem: The Magnes Press, 1993), 126-127. The *ḵātim* of Solomon in the *1001 Nights* is probably the Arabic equivalent of this phrase.

35 For example, the supposed western form is not attested in Federico Corriente, *A Dictionary of Andalusi Arabic* (Leiden: Brill, 1997).

36 Compare the Middle Persian term **mōm** 'wax' < Old Iranian *mauma* '*impure liquid*' – see Desmond Durkin-Meisterernst, *Dictionary of Manichaean Middle Persian and Parthian* (Turnhout: Brepols, 2004), 233; see also David N. MacKenzie, 'Mani's **Šābuhragān**,' *Bulletin of the School of Oriental and African Studies* 42 (1979): 531.

37 For my more detailed discussion of this term, see Siam Bhayro, "The Reception of Galen's Art of Medicine in the Syriac Book of Medicines", in B. Zipser (ed.), *Medical Books in the Byzantine World* (Bologna: Eikasmos Online II).

One would have thought that, if Simon was truly accessing Arabic sources like ar-Rāzī and Ibn Sīnā for himself, he would have been aware of their discussions of this term.[38]

Further Evidence for Simon's Use of Written and Oral Sources

It appears safe to say, therefore, that we have good reason to be skeptical about Simon's own knowledge of Arabic. It is clear that he is not only heavily reliant on Latin translations but he is also unable to utilize his own knowledge of Arabic to resolve the problems posed by them.

In addition to Latin translations of the Arabic texts, another written source utilized by Simon is the *Liber de doctrina arabica*, which was apparently a Latin lexicon of Arabic terminology. It must have proved very helpful, as Simon mentions it many times. The forms listed in the *Liber de doctrina arabica* are clearly MA – for example, see the discussion of *harxos* in **(w)** and the following:

(v) *Gemus arabice bubalus liber de doctrina arabica.*
Gemus is the Arabic word for Latin *bubalus* ('buffalo') according to the Arabic textbook.

CA   جَامُوسٌ   *jāmūsun* (L 455) > *jāmūs* > *jēmūs*

At this point, we are unable to identify the book. Nor can we tell whether it contained only Arabic and Latin terms, or whether it belonged to the tradition of more complex lists of *materia medica*.[39] As things stand, we can only go as far as to say that, given that the main centers for Arabic-Latin scholarship at the time were Italy[40] and Spain,[41] we should probably situate Simon's scholarly endeavors in a purely occidental context.

---

38 See also Charles Burnett's discussion of *Q littera* in this volume.

39 Cf., for example, the twelfth century **Kitāb al-Mustaʿīnī** by Ibn Baklarish, which contains Arabic, Syriac, Persian, Greek, Latin, Berber, Coptic and Romance terminology – see Charles Burnett (ed.), *Ibn Baklarish's Book of Simples: Medical Remedies between Three Faiths in Twelfth-Century Spain* (Oxford: The Arcadian Library in association with Oxford University Press, 2008).

40 E.g. Salerno – see Gerhard Baader, "Die Schule von Salerno", *Medizinhistorisches Journal* 13 (1978): 124-145.

41 E.g. Toledo – see Charles Burnett, "The Coherence of the Arabic-Latin Translation Program in Toledo in the Twelfth Century", *Science in Context* 14 (2001): 249-288.

As well as these written sources, Simon appears to have had at least three oral sources, i.e. either a colleague or native informants with whom he could consult:[42]

> **(w)** *Harsas arabice vel harxof quod melius est secundum Iudeum species cardi, cunchar vero species eius, verum in libro de doctrina arabica harxos est ipse cardus.*
> The Arabic *harsas*, or *harxof*, which is better according to Iudaeus, is a type of thistle, whereas *cunchar* is a type of thistle, but according to the Arabic textbook *harxos* means thistle itself.

CA   خَرْشَفٌ   *ḥaršafun* (D I.271, 'artichaut')

In example **(w)**, we would expect something like *ḥaršafun* > *ḥaršaf* (assuming that progressive vowel assimilation impedes *imāla* in the second syllable). It appears that Simon has two written sources at his disposal, both in Latin, and both showing the confusion between *f* and *s* that is common in Latin manuscripts (hence *harsas* and *harxos*).

In contrast to the preceding examples, in which Simon is not able to resolve the problems posed by his Latin sources, in this case he has some extra help. Indeed, it is clear that Simon's most reliable source regarding this term is Iudaeus,[43] who, in this case, is probably Abraham of Tortosa. It has often been noted that Simon and Abraham collaborated on a translation of az-Zahrāwī's *at-Taṣrīf li-man ʿajiza ʿan at-taʾlīf* 'The Arrangement of Medical Knowledge for the one who is not able to compile a book for himself' from Arabic into Latin, perhaps based on an already existing Hebrew translation.[44] It is not improbable, therefore, that Abraham, coming from the learned Iberian tradition of Arabic, Hebrew, and Latin scholarship, remained a valuable oral source for Simon as he compiled his *Clavis*.

---

42 For Simon's two female, native Arabic-speaking informants, see Zipser in this volume.

43 Iudaeus's *harxof* reflects a velarisation of š > x, with an accompanying shift a > o, which could suggest spoken rather than written transmission.

44 See, for example, Joseph Shatzmiller, *Jews, Medicine, and Medieval Society* (Berkeley and Los Angeles: University of California Press, 1994), 45; see also Ullmann, *Die Medizin*, 283.

Conclusion – Simon as 'Postmodernist'?

This raises one important question about Simon's method, namely its eclectic nature. In example **(w)**, we have a case where one of the three given forms is correct, while the other two are corrupted.[45] It is clearly not possible that all three are correct, so why did Simon not make a decision, omit the incorrect forms, and simply give the correct one? Simon's method is all the more startling on account of Iudaeus's correct identification being available to him.

   This very much suggests that Simon is not so much composing a dictionary in the modern sense, i.e. from an authoritative position with determinate meanings *etc.*, but rather simply compiling a group of sources into one work – i.e. producing what would be called today a 'postmodern' dictionary. In his discussion of this 'postmodern' approach to lexicography, which was used for the *Dictionary of Classical Hebrew*, David Clines wrote, 'Faced on many occasions, for example, with decisions about what data we should select and what we should compress, we have found ourselves concluding that there is no way of predicting which pieces of information will prove interesting and important to which users. So we have consistently regarded our task as providing and organizing the data that others will use as they think best, rather than imposing our own views as to what is significant'.[46] At first glance, it would appear that Simon is using a similar approach.

   We should not think that Simon has fortuitously stumbled upon this more 'progressive' method, however, as it is probably due to his inability to engage with the Arabic sources, which in turn compelled him to rely on a range of Latin sources and thus introduce errors and uncertainties into his *Clavis*.

---

45 There is some disagreement amongst the manuscripts regarding the final *harxos* but, whichever reading is preferred, we are still left with at least one corrupt form (i.e. the initial *harsas*) and one correct form (*harxof*) – the following point is valid either way.

46 David J. A. Clines (ed.), *The Dictionary of Classical Hebrew: Volume I* (Sheffield: Sheffield Academic Press, 1993), 26.

Bibliography

Baader, Gerhard. "Die Schule von Salerno," *Medizinhistorisches Journal* 13 (1978): 124-145.

Bhayro, Siam. "The Reception of Galen's Art of Medicine in the Syriac Book of Medicines." in B. Zipser (ed.), *Medical Books in the Byzantine World*. Bologna: Eikasmos Online II.

Blau, Joshua. *A Grammar of Christian Arabic based mainly on South Palestinian Texts from the First Millennium.* 3 vols. Louvain: CSCO, 1966.

— "Some Observations on a Middle Arabic Egyptian Text in Coptic Characters." *Jerusalem Studies in Arabic and Islam* 1 (1979): 215-262.

— "The State of Research in the Field of the Linguistic Study of Middle Arabic." *Arabica* 28 (1981): 187-203.

— *The Emergence and Linguistic Background of Judaeo-Arabic: A Study of the Origins of Neo-Arabic and Middle Arabic.* 3rd revised edition; Jerusalem: Ben-Zvi Institute, 1999.

— *A Handbook of Early Middle Arabic.* Jerusalem: The Max Schloessinger Memorial Foundation, 2002.

Burnett, Charles. "The Coherence of the Arabic-Latin Translation Program in Toledo in the Twelfth Century." *Science in Context* 14 (2001): 249-288.

Burnett, Charles (ed.). *Ibn Baklarish's Book of Simples: Medical Remedies between Three Faiths in Twelfth-Century Spain.* Oxford: The Arcadian Library in association with Oxford University Press, 2008.

Clines, David J. A. (ed.). *The Dictionary of Classical Hebrew.* Volume I. Sheffield: Sheffield Academic Press, 1993.

Corriente, Federico. *A Dictionary of Andalusi Arabic.* Leiden: Brill, 1997.

den Heijer, Johannes. "Introduction: Middle and Mixed Arabic, a New Trend in Arabic Studies," in Liesbeth Zack and Arie Schippers (Eds), *Middle Arabic and Mixed Arabic: Diachrony and Synchrony.* 1-25. Leiden: Brill, 2012.

Dozy, Reinhart. *Supplément aux Dictionnaires Arabes*, 2 vols; Leiden: Brill, 1881.

Durkin-Meisterernst, Desmond. *Dictionary of Manichaean Middle Persian and Parthian.* Turnhout: Brepols, 2004.

Hopkins, Simon. *Studies in the Grammar of Early Arabic based upon Papyri Datable to before A.H. 300/A.D. 912.* Oxford: Oxford University Press, 1984.

Lane, Edward William. *An Arabic-English Lexicon,* Parts 1-8 and Supplement; London: Williams and Norgate, 1863-1893.

MacKenzie, David N. "Mani's Šābuhragān." *Bulletin of the School of Oriental and African Studies* 42 (1979): 500-534.

Naveh, Joseph and Shaul Shaked. *Magic Spells and Formulae: Aramaic Incantations of Late Antiquity.* Jerusalem: The Magnes Press, 1993.

Pormann, Peter E. and Emilie Savage-Smith. *Medieval Islamic Medicine.* Edinburgh: Edinburgh University Press, 2007.

Shatzmiller, Joseph. Jews, *Medicine, and Medieval Society.* Berkeley and Los Angeles: University of California Press, 1994.

Ullmann, Manfred. *Die Medizin im Islam.* Leiden: Brill, 1970.

Versteegh, Kees. *The Arabic Language.* Edinburgh: Edinburgh University Press, 1997.

Wright, William. *A Grammar of the Arabic Language,* translated from the German of Caspari and edited with numerous additions and corrections. 3rd edition revised by W. Robertson Smith and M. J. de Goeje; 2 vols. Cambridge: Cambridge University Press, 1951.

Edited by **Barbara Zipser**

Charles Burnett (Warburg Institute)

Simon of Genoa's Use of the *Breviarium* of Stephen, the Disciple of Philosophy

Among the sources most frequently cited by Simon of Genoa in his *Clavis sanationis*, is 'Ste.' or 'Stephanus' sometimes with the addition '*in synonimis*' or even '*in suis synonimis*'. Altogether there are over 385 citations of this kind. It was Moritz Steinschneider[1] who first guessed that this 'Stephanus' might be Stephen, 'the disciple of philosophy', who translated the *Regalis dispositio* or *Liber completus* of Haly Abbas ('Ali ibn al-'Abbas al-Majusi) in 1127. But he was a bit perplexed by the fact that the glossary clearly marked '*synonyma*', which accompanied the printed versions of the *Regalis dispositio*, was clearly not Stephen's, but was none other than a version of Simon of Genoa's *Clavis sanationis*, which the Renaissance editor presumptuously attributed to himself.[2] It was Valentin Rose who, when he described the manuscripts of the Staatsbibliothek (at that time, Königliche Bibliothek) in Berlin fourteen years later (1905), discovered a manuscript of Haly Abbas which ended with Stephen's own glossary.[3] Because of *verbatim* correspondence with the *Clavis sanationis* (examples of which he provided), Rose was convinced that this glossary was the 'Synonyma' of Stephen, even though it did not bear the title '*synonyma*', but rather '*breviarium*'. This article will consider more closely the relationship between Simon's *Clavis sanationis* and Stephen's *Breviarium*, using the printed edition of the *Clavis sanationis*,[4] the manuscript of the *Regalis dispositio* that Rose described: *MS lat. Fol. 74* (Rose no. 898 = **B**),[5] and another, contemporary, manuscript: Worcester, *Cathedral Library* F 40 (= **F**).

---

1 Moritz Steinschneider, "Zur Literatur der Synonyma." In J.L. Pagel (Ed.) *Leben. Lehre und Leistungen des Heinrich von Mondeville (Hermondaville), 1. Die Chirurgie des Heinrich von Mondeville (Hermondaville)*. (Berlin: Hirschwald, 1892), 582-595.

2 Haly filius Abbas, *Liber totius medicine... (Regalis dispositio)*, Lyons, 1523, f. 1r: "*Synonyma de pluribus medicinae autoribus a magistro Michaele de Capella, artium et medicinae doctore, collecta, huic libro Hali Abbatis de regali dispositione perutili*" ('The synonyms collected from many authorities in medicine by Master Michael de Capella, a doctor of Arts and Medicine, being very useful for this book of Haly Abbas on *The Royal Arrangement*').

3 Valentin Rose, *Verzeichniss der lateinischen Handschriften der Königlichen Bibliothek zu Berlin*, II.3. (Berlin: Behrend, 1905), 1059-1065.

4 As available on '*Simon Online*' (www.simonofgenoa.org).

5 The first part of this copy of the *Regalis dispositio* is now MS Leipzig, *Univ. bibl.*, 1131.

Let us first look at Stephen's text. The *Regalis dispositio* consists of ten books of medical theory and ten books of medical practice. Stephen already promised, at the end of his preface to the second, practical part of the work, to include a breviary of all the *materia medica* in Dioscorides:

Nec vero omnino lectorem errori et sollicitudini remisimus, set quod posse nobis fuit et Oriens habebat, in totius operis fine omnium que apud Diascoridem sunt medicaminum breviarium subdidimus, hinc eorum nomina Grece, illinc Arabice habens, ut in cuius venerit hoc opus manus, quid queque res sit aut Grecum si invenit aut certe Arabem, sit illi posse consulere. Reliqua vero, que Arabica sunt tantum, aut propriis protulimus diffinitionibus, que quidem potuimus, aut omnino siluimus, studium daturi ut si quovis modo nobis posse gratia dederit divina, inter Greca et Arabica nomina inseramus Latina.

We have not altogether consigned the reader to error and worry, but added at the end of the whole work what we could do, and what the Orient could provide: [namely] a breviary of all the *materia medica* in Dioscorides, on this side giving the names in Greek, on that side in Arabic. Thus, in whoever's hands this work arrives, he can consult a Greek, if he finds one, or indeed an Arab, about what each thing is. The [names] which are only in Arabic, we have either put forward with their proper definitions, when we were able to do so, or we have been silent about them, intending to make an effort to insert the Latin names among the Greek and Arabic ones, if Divine Grace gives us any possibility to do this.[6]

Similar sentiments are included in Stephen's short preface to the *Breviarium* itself, which runs as follows:

Ad umbilicum, per Dei gratiam, nostre translationis deducto labore, quod reliquum est quodque in huius secunde partis polliciti sumus principiis, medicaminum omnium breviarium subdimus, quod, collatis et Arabice et Grece scriptis Diascoridis libris, elucubrati iunctamus ut, quoniam Latinorum nobis nominum ad liquidum peritia non est, qui ad nostrum accesserit opus studiosus lector, de incognitis quos possit consulere habeat. Nam et in Sicilia et Salerni, ubi horum maxime studiosi sunt, et Greci habentur et lingue gnari Arabice, quos qui voluerit

---

6 An edition, with manuscript variants, of this preface is given in Charles Burnett, "Antioch as a Link between Arabic and Latin Culture in the Twelfth and Thirteenth Centuries." in Anne Tihon, Isabelle Draelants and Baudouin van den Abeele (Eds.) *Occident et Proche-Orient: contacts scientifiques au temps des croisades.* (Turnhout: Brepols, 2000), 1-78 (see 37-38). Reprinted with corrections in Charles Burnett, "Antioch as a Link between Arabic and Latin Culture in the Twelfth and Thirteenth Centuries." in Charles Burnett (ed.), *Arabic into Latin in the Middle Ages: The Translators and their Intellectual and Social Context.* (Farnham: Ashgate Variorum, 2009), Article IV.

consulere poterit. Et Greca quidem nomina ut sunt plane exponimus, quippe qui eisdem fere in sono utimur quibus et illi elementis, Arabica non sic, cum apud illos quedam sint littere quarum omnino Latina extorris est lingua. Scripsimus itaque illa vicinioribus quibus potuimus. Iam ergo hinc propositum incipiamus.

Having brought to an end, thanks be to God, the labour of our translation, we shall add what remains to be done and what we promised at the beginning of this second part: [namely] a breviary of all the *materia medica*. Having toiled over this by comparing the books of Dioscorides written in both Arabic and Greek, since our experience of the Latin names is not firm, we enjoin any studious reader who takes up our work, to seek out those whom he can consult over those names unknown to him. For both in Sicily and in Salerno, where especially there are students of these matters, there are both Greeks and people who know the Arabic language, whom anyone can consult at his will. The Greek words we write clearly, just as they are, since we use letters that are almost the same in sound as those they use. It is not so, however, for the Arabic words, since among them there are certain letters to which the Latin language is completely alien. Thus we have represented them with the closest letters possible. Let us now begin from here.[7]

The glossary immediately follows. In the Berlin manuscript the Greek terms are written on the left hand side of the page, the Arabic terms on the right, and the occasional Latin terms in the middle (**Figure 1**); they fill eighteen pages. In the Worcester manuscript the scribe attempts to cram the whole glossary into four pages, using four columns, and then six columns, to get everything in, and marking the columns of Greek and Arabic words with alternate red and turquoise vertical lines. There are some 575 items altogether—in Latin transliteration, but arranged in strict Greek alphabetical order. Stephen mentions Dioscorides as a name that would have been well known to his Latin audience. However, he shows no dependence on any Latin translation of the *De re medica*, and this is not surprising. The early (sixth-century) translation of *De re medica* was not widely copied, and the 'Constantinian' revision of this work was hardly beginning to make an impact in 1127 (its first manuscripts are from the twelfth century).[8] If he had known either of these versions he probably would have disregarded them as being inaccurate and lacunose (as he did in respect to

---

[7] Burnett, "Antioch as a Link …", 2009, 38-39.

[8] John M. Riddle, "Dioscorides." in F. Edward Cranz and Paul Oscar Kristeller (Eds.). *Catalogus translationum et commentariorum*, IV, (Washington: Catholic Univ. of America Pr., 1980), 1-143.

Constantine the African's earlier translation of the *Regalis dispositio*).[9] Rather, it is clear that he used Greek and Arabic texts directly (as he claimed). The *De re medica* had been rearranged according to a strict alphabetical order early in the Greek transmission of the text.[10] Stephen is evidently transliterating a Greek text, rather than an Arabic text that preserved the Greek in transliteration. This is obvious from the consistency in which he transliterates the Greek letters. In keeping with Byzantine pronunciation ioticization is present throughout,[11] the rough breathing ('h') is omitted, and non-initial *beta*, when followed by a vowel or 'r' becomes a fricative. No difference is made between long and short vowels, and double consonants are usually represented as single. 'Ai' (*alpha iota*) is written 'ae' initially and 'e' within words, *theta* as 'th', and *kappa* usually as a 'k' (and always as 'k' as an initial; but 'k', 'c', 'qu' occur within words). 'X' is used for *khi*, which could be a simple taking-over of the Greek letter. Greek *xi* is 'cs', just as *psi* is 'ps'.

In the right-hand column appear the Arabic transcriptions. Here, the transcription of the consonants is less rigorous: no differentiation is made between *qaf* and *kaf*, for which 'c' and 'qu' are used interchangeably, between *sin, shin,* and *sad*, all of which are transliterated as 's', and *dal* and *dhal* which are both 'd'. There is variation in the two manuscripts between transliterating *jim* as 'g' or as 'i', while *ʿayn* is usually represented by an 'h' (occasionally by an 'a'). No special letters have been used. This perhaps reflects a spoken Arabic, rather than the written language, and this might explain the intercalation of vowels within consonant clusters, and the *imala* ('e' for 'a' and even 'i' for long 'u'). But Stephen is consistent in not assimilating the definite article to the following consonant (*al-* is always written 'el-') and, occasionally, errors suggest a misreading of Arabic script.[12] As he says himself in the preface to the second part of the *Regalis dispositio*, he assimilates the Arabic words to Latin morphology, making them either neuter words, ending in '–um', or feminine, ending in '–a', and declining

---

9 For his sharp criticism of Constantine's earlier translation of the *Regalis dispositio* of ʿAli ibn al-ʿAbbas al-Majusi (*Pantegni*), see Charles Burnett "The Legend of Constantine the African", *Micrologus. Natura, scienze e società medievali / Nature, Sciences and Medieval Societies* 21 (2013), 277–94.

10 I owe a great debt to Marie Cronier for recognising that Stephen's index belongs to the Syro-Palestinian family of the Greek Dioscorides, among which the manuscript Florence, Laur. plut. 74.23, gives a similar index, edited by Max Wellmann in Dioscorides (1906-1914), III, 109-135.

11 *Upsilon* is usually written 'u', but presumably would have been pronounced as a front vowel (as in French 'u'), since it is differentiated by Stephen from 'ou'.

12 E.g. 'zague' is written for 'raghwa' and 'zirum' for 'ziz' (the letters *ra* and *za* differ by only one dot); 'defifum' is written for 'daqiq' and 'bereniasecum' for 'birinjasaf' (*qaf* and *fa* differ by only one dot).

them as necessary.[13] This implies that it is the Arabic terms that Stephen and his colleagues are accustomed to using, and this impression is corroborated by the fact that, when adjectives or qualifying nouns are added to the term, they are in Latin ('*agrestis*' = 'wild', '*sanguis*' = 'the blood of', and colour adjectives).[14] Contrary to what is implied at the end of the preface to the second part, there are no Arabic words without Greek equivalents.

As for Latin equivalents, sometimes they are only the Latin spellings of the Greek words (ending in '*–um*' rather than '*–on*'). At other times they are of native Latin origin; in no case is a Romance form (whether *lingua franca* or Italian) given. Glosses in Latin, however, often provide a complement or a substitute for a translation: the Greek '*adarkes*' is translated as '*spuma cannarum*', with a gloss in Latin 'which sticks to reed-canes'; *defifum* is described as 'a certain porridge that is made' (no Latin equivalent is given); '*androseimon*' is not translated but the phrase is added: '*Dicit Iohannes esse dadiam masculam, id est pellis ubi conduntur testiculi*' ('John says that it is 'masculine *dadia*, i.e. the skin under which the testicles are hidden'); and '*bekhion*' is described as '*herba que a tusse denominatur*' ('the herb which is named from coughing'). In only one case is there a reference to the 'common people': '*vocat vulgus*' ('the people call') the blood of the chameleon '*camelum iudeacum*'.

Stephen ends the glossary with a reiteration of the fact that he has used only Greek and Arabic sources:

> *Hec sunt que in Siria ad presens nostra invenit manus de medicaminum interpretatione Grece et Arabice. In quo si quid erratum posteritas invenerit, nobis non imputandum credat. Neque enim noster est set aliorum labor, et sic inventum posuimus. Si autem dederit Deus et otium gerendorum affuerit, utrumque plenius rimaturi sumus.*
>
> These are what our hand found concerning the interpretation of *materia medica* in Greek and Arabic. If posterity finds anything wrong in this, it should not be blamed on us. For it is not our work, but rather that of others, and we have just put it forward as we found it. But if God allows us, and we have the leisure to do so, we shall explore each [Greek and Arabic] more fully.[15]

---

13 Burnett, "Antioch as a Link ...", 2009, 35-36: *quoniam... omnia... hic fere posita medicaminum nomina Arabum proferuntur lingua, et nos Latina parum habebamus assueta, prout sunt in Arabico, ea proferimus, etiam que cognita nobis sunt nonnumquam, que incognita ubique, set ad Latine formam declinationis inclinata.* Since... almost all the names of the medicaments here [in Haly Abbas's book] are presented in the language of the Arabs, and we are little accustomed to the Latin names, we present them as they are in Arabic—sometimes even those which are known to us; in all cases when they are unknown to us, but we decline them according to the Latin.

14 This also agrees with Stephen's policy for simple medicines in the text of Haly Abbas, where he retains the Arabic forms in Latin transcription, with Latin terminations (see below).

15 Burnett "Antioch as a Link ...", 2009, 39-40.

So, it is clear that Stephen, the Disciple of Philosophy, had access to Dioscorides' *De re medica*, in Greek as well as to an Arabic translation, if not to a text in which the Arabic terms were already listed alongside the Greek.[16] This access was in Antioch (he mentions 'Siria'), where we know that the books of the *Regalis dispositio* were translated (or at least copied) at various dates within 1127.[17]

We know from another translation he made—the *Book of the Configuration of the World* (within the *Liber Mamonis*), a cosmology by Ibn al-Haytham—that Stephen was an excellent translator, with a very high level of knowledge of both the language and the subject matter,[18] and the *Breviarium* witnesses to a similar level of diligence and competence.

✳

What did Simon of Genoa make of Stephen's *Breviarium*? First of all, it must be stated that, in the preface to the *Clavis sanationis*, where he gives a detailed list of all the authorities on which he bases his work, he fails to mention the name of Stephen and his glossary completely. Admittedly, Simon does not mention *any* Latin author or translator more recent than the eleventh-century Gariopontus (the *Passionarius*), and passes over in silence any debt that he may have had to more recent medical writers. But it does seem a little strange that Stephen features so prominently in the *Clavis* itself, but receives no comment in the preface. On the other hand Simon refers to Haly Abbas's *Liber completus*, without mentioning that Stephen is the translator. He makes some rather uncomplimentary remarks concerning the book:

---

16 Abu Bakr Muhammad ibn Zakariyya' al-Razi refers to texts on *materia medica* 'in three columns: a column for Greek, a column for Syriac, and one for Arabic' (Emilie Savage-Smith, "The Working Files of Rhazes: Are the Jami' and the Hawi Identical?" in Rotraud Hansberger, M. Afifi al-Akiti and Charles Burnett (Eds.), *Medieval Arabic Thought: Essays in Honour of Fritz Zimmermann.* (London, Turin: Warburg Institute, 2012), 173.

17 As a typical example, one may quote the statement at the beginning of the eighth book of the second part of Haly filius Abbas, *Liber totius medicine*....Lyons, 1523, f. 261v: *Translatio Stephani phylosophie discipuli de Arabico in Latinum scripsitque ipse et complevit anno a passione Domini millesimo centesimo vicesimo .vii. mense Novembris die .iii. feria septima apud Antiochiam*. The translation from Arabic into Latin of Stephen, the disciple of philosophy. He wrote the copy himself and completed it in the year from the passion of our Lord 1127, on Saturday, November the third, at Antioch.

18 This is the subject of a thesis being completed at the Warburg Institute, University of London, by Dirk Grupe, "The Latin reception of Arabic astronomy and cosmology in mid-twelfth-century Antioch: The Liber Mamonis and the Dresden Almagest", unpublished PhD thesis, University of London, 2013.

Et ex libro Aliabatis qui vocatur liber completus in quo admodum parum proficere potui. Nam vocabulorum que continet quedam neque Greca neque Arabica sunt, et aliqua Greca et aliqua Arabica, sed ad Latinum modum declinandi extorta et ob hoc a propria prolatione corrupta.

I also used the book of Haly Abbas, which is called the 'Complete Book' from which I was able to draw very little profit. For, of the words that it contains, some are neither Greek nor Arabic; others are Greek and Arabic but have been twisted into the Latin way of declining, and because of this their proper pronunciation has been corrupted.[19]

These statements are borne out by the use Simon makes of Haly Abbas, and his comments on the work, in the body of the *Clavis*. There are only some twenty-four references to the text, either as 'Haly/Ali (with or without 'Abbatis')', or as '*Regalis dispositio*' (never '*liber completus*'), or as both – which counts as 'profiting very little'. And we find comments such as:

In regali vero dispositione Hali vocatur bululengeri, sed nec Grecum neque Arabicum est.
In the *Regalis Dispositio* of Haly it is called '*bululengeri*', but it is neither Greek nor Arabic. *Ezeledari in secundo pratice Aliab. exponitur quod est zinziber nec Grecum nec Arabicum est.*
Ezeledari in the second [book] of the *Practica* is explained as being ginger, but it is neither Greek nor Arabic.[20]

The 'second book of the *Practica*' referred to here and in several other references to Haly, is the book of the *Regalis dispositio* which is devoted to medical simples *(materia medica)*, of which, from chapter thirty-four onwards, it gives an annotated list. As such it is sometimes called the *Antidotarium*. Most of Simon's quotations from the *Regalis dispositio* seem to come from this source. 'Bullulengeri' happens to be the first item in this list:

Bullulengeri (i.e. absinthium B in marg.) excellentior huius species est croceum, novum in quo sit pauca ponticitas et quod aufertur de regione Sirie in partibus Tarsi (in rasi pr). Eius complexio calida est in primo gradu, sicca in tertio, sapor eius amarus...
Bullulengeri the best of this species is yellow and fresh, in which there is a little tartness, and what is taken from the region of Syria in the area of Tarsus. Its complexion is hot in the first degree, dry in the third, its taste is bitter...[21]

---

19 *Clavis*, Preface §4.
20 Ibid., *Abscintium, Ezeledari*.
21 Haly filius Abbas, *Liber totius medicine... (Regalis dispositio)*, Lyons, 1523, f. 166r, MS B, fol.

The references to the *Regalis dispositio* are distinguished from those to '*Stephanus*' (with or without the mention of '*synonima*'):

> *Saber vel sabr Ara<bice> est aloes, apud Aliab<as> invenitur sabare et in syno<nimis> Step<hani> sabarum.*
> Sabar or sabr in Arabic is aloes. In Haly Abbas is found '*sabare*' and in the Synonyms of Stephen '*sabarum*'.
> *Ste<phanus> etiam in suis synonimis dicit quod anagallus est auricula muris... S<tephanus> in synonimis de M. et in secundo pratice Hali.*
> Stephen also in his *Synonyms* says that '*anagallus*' is mouse-ear... under 'm', and in the second [book] of the *Practica* of Haly.[22]

Nevertheless, Simon clearly knew that Stephen had translated the *Regalis dispositio*. For, at the beginning of his account of the *materia medica* beginning with 'q' he writes:

> *Q littera nec Greci nec Arabes habent. Stephanus tamen translator Regalis dispositionis multa vocabula que per chef vel kaf scribuntur apud Arabes per q scripsit.*
> Neither the Greeks nor the Arabs have the letter 'q'. Stephen, the translator of the *Regalis dispositio*, however, wrote many words that are written with a *qaf* or *kaf* in Arabic, with a 'q'.[23]

An indication that Simon had the *Breviarium* in front of him when describing the *Synonima,* is his statement that:

> *Idem error apparet in synonimis Ste<phani> ubi nomina G<reca> exponuntur per A<rabica>, deinde per Latina.*
> The same error appears in the *Synonyms* of Stephen, where Greek names are explained through Arabic ones, and then through Latin names.[24]

Simon's use of the *Breviarium* is corroborated from the more extensive quotations from the *Synonima*:

---

22 *Clavis, Saber* and *Auricula muris.*
23 Ibid., *Q littera.*
24 Ibid., *Nux romana.*

CLAVIS SANATIONIS	BREVIARIUM
Ste<phanus> in Synonimis agalosia est xiloaloes ab India veniens (s. v. agalugim)	agaloxon (Gr.) xiloaloes (Lat.) aud (Ar.) quod ab India aufertur
alupum exponit Ste<phanus> quod est terbedum et est turbith (s.v. alupum)	alupon (Gr.) turbit (Lat.) terbedum (Ar.)
atriplex G<rece> vocatur andrafaxis apud D<iascuridem> ... sed Ara<bice> kataf et sarmeth dicitur, Ste<fanus> coatutum et sermach (s.v. atriplex)	andrafaxis (Gr.) atriplex (Lat.) sermacum catafum (Ar.)
adharcis... Ste<fanus> in synonimis adharsis vel adarchion, et est spuma que circa cannas adunatur (s.v. adharcis)	adarkis vel adarchion (Gr.) spuma cannarum (Lat.) zague (Ar. = raghwa) que circa cannas adunatur
aethyopis Ste<phanus>: est specie busami et cinami ab epythopia (s.v. aethyopis)	aethiopis (Gr.) – (Lat.) species busim (Ar.) et est ei nomen ab Ethiopia
asum Ste.: pro as scripsit: quod est mirtus Arabice (s.v. asum)	mursini (Gr.) mirtus (Lat.) assum (Ar.)

One can see immediately from these comparisons that Simon's version is considerably corrupt in respect to the original. That this is not entirely the fault of the condition of the text of the *Clavis sanationis* is clear from Simon's own statements concerning the faultiness of Stephen's terms:

> *Ageratos ... Ste[phanus] in synonimis exposuit per Arabicum helfa, quod ignoro.*
> Stephen explains this through the Arabic word *helfa*, which I do not recognize.
> *Aedyonela exponit [.g.] Ste. per Arabicum cadite leiel utrumque ignoro.*
> Stephen explains *Aedyonela* through the Arabic *cadite leiel*, both of which I do not recognize.
> *Asmachum dixit Ste<phanus> vocari absinthium sed nescio qua lingua.*
> Stephen has said that *absinthe* is called *asmachum*, but I do not know in what language.[25]

When one looks at the manuscripts of the *Breviarium*, the words become much clearer. We find '*Aedionelafu*', which is the literal transliteration of αἰδοῖον ἐλάφου, for which the Arabic equivalent is '*cadit eleiel*' in which 't' has been written in place of 'b': *qadib al-ayyil*. Both terms mean 'deer's penis'. '*Asmachum*' is simply a corruption, since the manuscripts of the *Breviarium* clearly give the Greek transliteration '*absinthion*' (ἀψίνθιον) and the Arabic transliteration '*afsinthin*' (B)/*absinthiï* (F).

In many cases Simon simply points out that Stephen has added a Latin ending to the word ('*assum*' for '*as*', '*basalum*' for '*basal*', etc.). Typical is 'Stephanus has written x for y', such as '*Bablegum scripsit Ste. pro belilico.*'[26]

---

25 Ibid., *Ageratos, Aedyonela, Asmachum.*
26 Ibid., *Bablegum.*

It is evident, therefore, that Simon had access to a text of Stephen's *Breviarium* which was considerably corrupted. What remains to be done is to trace the route by which the *Breviarium* of Stephen, the Disciple of Philosophy, an incomplete but competent piece of work, became the *Synonyma* of Stephen, and in the process of transmission became corrupted into the form known to Simon of Genoa.

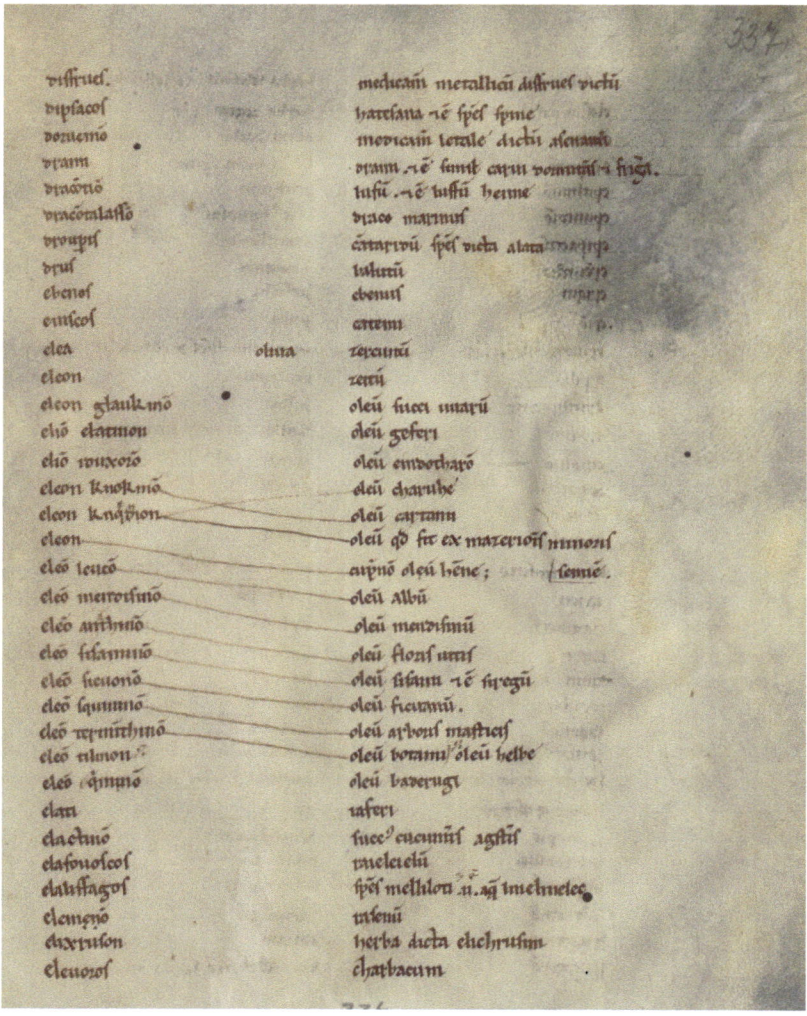

Figure 1. Staatsbibliothek zu Berlin, Preussischer Kulturbesitz, *lat. fol.* 74, ff. 334v

Bibliography

Burnett, Charles. "Antioch as a Link between Arabic and Latin Culture in the Twelfth and Thirteenth Centuries." In Anne Tihon, Isabelle Draelants and Baudouin van den Abeele (Eds.) *Occident et Proche-Orient: contacts scientifiques au temps des croisades*. 1–78. Turnhout: Brepols, 2000.

— "Antioch as a Link between Arabic and Latin Culture in the Twelfth and Thirteenth Centuries." In Charles Burnett (Ed.) *Arabic into Latin in the Middle Ages: The Translators and their Intellectual and Social Context*. Farnham: Ashgate Variorum, 2009, Article IV.

— "The Legend of Constantine the African." *Micrologus. Natura, scienze e società medievali / Nature, Sciences and Medieval Societies* 21 (2013): 277–94.

Dioscorides *De materia medica, libri quinque*, ed. Max Wellmann, 3 vol. Berlin: Weidmann, 1906-1914.

Grupe, Dirk. "The Latin reception of Arabic astronomy and cosmology in mid-twelfth-century Antioch: The Liber Mamonis and the Dresden Almagest", unpublished PhD thesis, University of London, 2013.

Riddle, John M. "Dioscorides." In F. Edward Cranz and Paul Oscar Kristeller (Eds.). *Catalogus translationum et commentariorum*, IV. 1-143. Washington: Catholic Univ. of America Pr., 1980.

Rose, Valentin. *Verzeichniss der lateinischen Handschriften der Königlichen Bibliothek zu Berlin*, II.3. 1059-1065. Berlin: Behrend, 1905.

Savage-Smith, Emilie. "The Working Files of Rhazes: Are the Jamiʿ and the Hawi Identical?" In Rotraud Hansberger, M. Afifi al-Akiti and Charles Burnett (Eds.) *Medieval Arabic Thought: Essays in Honour of Fritz Zimmermann*. 163-180. London, Turin: Warburg Institute, 2012.

Steinschneider, Moritz. "Zur Literatur der Synonyma." In Julius Leopold Pagel (Ed.) *Leben. Lehre und Leistungen des Heinrich von Mondeville (Hermondaville), 1. Die Chirurgie des Heinrich von Mondeville (Hermondaville).* 582-595. Berlin: Hirschwald, 1892.

Marie Cronier

Dioscorides Excerpts in Simon of Genoa's *Clavis sanationis*

The Greek pharmacologist Dioscorides (*floruit* during the second half of the first century AD) is one of the most frequently quoted authors in Simon of Genoa's *Clavis sanationis*. Simon also makes a statement to this effect in his *Praefatio* (§ 4), when he says: '*Primum ex grecis Dyas*[*coridis*] *liber producatur*', Among the Greeks, one must first refer to Dioscorides' book:[1] thus, Simon considers Dioscorides' treatise as the first and the most important.

This work Simon refers to is nowadays commonly referred to by its Latin title *De materia medica*, although it was written in Greek (Περὶ ὕλης ἰατρικῆς/Peri hylēs iatrikēs): it is a large encyclopedia of pharmacology, containing about eight hundred chapters, each of which being dedicated to one specific 'simple' (a plant, a vegetable, an animal, a metal, *etc.*).

1. General Remarks

It must first be stressed that Simon never seems to refer to other Greek treatises attributed to Dioscorides (*Euporista, Alexipharmaca,* or *Theriaca*), which are most probably apocryphal and, in any case, are not known through late antique or medieval Latin translations.

Usually, moreover, Simon's quotations of Dioscorides are quite long and often consist of several sentences. He introduces them with different abbreviations ('*Dyascor.*' or '*Dya.*' or even a simple '*D.*'), which can be found very often in Simon's work. I have not yet made an exhaustive list of all these quotations but a brief survey suggests that there are several hundred. However, in some chapters where Dioscorides' name is not mentioned, it is in fact possible to find authentic quotations of *De materia medica*. This is the case, for example, of chapter '*Apios siue camebalanos*' (tuberous spurge), as can be observed:

---

1 In this paper, I will quote Simon's *Clavis sanationis* using the very useful online edition: http://www.simonofgenoa.org , with my own collations of the other witnesses, as proposed on this website. Translations are mine.

Apios. Siue camebalanos siue rafanus agrestis: astas habet duas uel tres, uiscosas et teneras et ruffas; folia sunt ei rute similia, longa uiridia et parua; fructus siue semen paruum; cuius radix est affodilo similis, obrotunda, similis pile, lacrimo plena, a foris nigra, intus alba; radices eius due sunt super terram et cetera.

1 *apios* AC: *appios* B f | *rafanus* ABC: *raffanus* f | *astas* ABC: *hastas* f | *duas* B: *quinque*
   AC : *duas* e : (unclear) f | *uiscosas* ACf: *iuntosas* B
2 *uiridia* ABf : *uirida* C
3 *obrotunda* AC : *et obrotunda* B f | *a foris* ABC : *foris* f |
4 *nigra* Af : *niger* B

Apios [tuberous spurge], or *camebalanos* or *rafanus agrestis* [wild radish]: it has two or three stems, sticky, thin and red. Its leaves are similar to those of the rue, long, pale-green and small. Its fruit or seed is small. Its root is similar to that of the asphodel, round, like a ball[2], full of juice, black from outside but white inside. It has two roots above the ground.[3]

Although Dioscorides' name does not appear, even in an abbreviated form, this chapter is obviously a translation of the original Greek chapter from *De materia medica* (book IV, chapter 175: ἄπιος/apios):[4]

ἄπιος · οἱ δὲ ἰσχάδα, οἱ δὲ χαμαιβάλανον, οἱ δὲ ῥάφανον ἀγρίαν, οἱ δὲ λινόζωστιν καλοῦσι. κλωνία δύο ἢ τρία ἀπὸ γῆς σχοινώδη, λεπτά, ἐρυθρά, μικρὸν ὑπὲρ τῆς γῆς αἴροντα· φύλλα πηγάνῳ ἐοικότα, ἐπιμηκέστερα <δέ>, χλωρά· καρπὸς μικρός· ῥίζα ἀσφοδέλῳ παραπλησία, στρογγυλωτέρα δὲ καὶ πρὸς τὸ τοῦ ἀπίου σχῆμα, μεστὴ ὀποῦ, φλοιὸν ἔχουσα ἔξωθεν μέλανα, ἔνδοθεν δὲ λευκή. The tuberous spurge: some people call it *ischas*, others *chamaibalanon*, others *rhaphanos agria*, and others *linozostis*. It sends up from the ground two or three stringy little twigs, thin, red, and rising slightly above ground. The leaves resemble those of the rue but they are longer and pale-green. The fruit is small. The root closely resembles that of the asphodel but it is rounder, tending toward being pear-shaped, full of milky juice, and it has skin that is black on the outside, but inside the root is white.

---

2 The altered form *'pile'* (*pila* has many significations, for example: ball) obviously comes from a confusion with *'pire'* (*pira*, pear), which is the correct form, cf. the Greek text.

3 The last sentence is probably the result of an alteration of some Greek words that had been omitted above, in the description of the stems: μικρὸν ὑπὲρ τῆς γῆς αἴροντα, *rising slightly above the ground* (cf. the Greek text).

4 The reference edition for the Greek text of *De materia medica* is: *Dioscorides De materia medica, libri quinque*, edited by Max Wellmann, 3 vol. (Berlin: Weidmann, 1906-1914. Reeditions: Berlin, 2010) (quoted in the following: Wellmann). The English translation quoted in this paper is: Pedanius Dioscorides of Anazarbus. *De materia medica*, translated by Lily Y. Beck. Altertumswissenschaftliche Texte und Studien 38. Hildesheim-Zürich-New York: Olms-Weidmann, 2005. For the identifications of the plants, I mainly rely on: Max Aufmesser, *Etymologische und wortgeschichtliche Erläuterungen zu De materia medica des Pedanius Dioscurides Anazarbeus.* (Hildesheim-Zürich-New York: Olms-Weidmann, 2000).

In a consequence, the chapters coming from Dioscorides in Simon's treatise are even more numerous than those who bear the attribution to this author.

Another fact to be underlined is that, in general, Simon only quotes the descriptive part of Dioscorides' chapter and totally omits the passages dealing with therapeutic properties. Thus, when a 'simple' is dealt with in the *De materia medica*, it is almost always quoted by Simon, except when Dioscorides does not give any description of it but only speaks about its therapeutic properties: in this case, Simon either resorts to another author or gives his own description.

2. Simon's Sources for Dioscorides in Latin

First, let us have a look at what Simon says in his *Praefatio*:

> *Primum ex grecis Dyascoridis liber producatur (...) Verum liber eius qui ab antiquo in latinum habetur a primo exemplari differt. Nam hic per alphabetum in latinum ordinatus est. Ille uero in V libris distinctus ut per ipsius prohemium demonstratur. Multa etiam capitula in hoc desunt que ille continet, aliqua etiam in hoc libro sunt addita, que ipsius auctoris non sunt: per Serapionem de simplicibus medicinis et per hoc opos ostenditur.*
>
> 1 *ex* ACf : *de* B | *Dyascoridis* C : *Dyas.* A, *Diascoridis* B, *Dy.* f |
> 2 *habetur – latinum om.* f | *in* AC : *om.* B
> 3. *libris* ABC : *libros* f
> 4. *capitula* ACf: *capitulla* B | *in hoc* ABC : *om.* f | *libro* ABC: *om.* f |
> 5. *auctoris* ABf : *auctore* C | *per* ABC: *ut per* f
> 6. *opos* AC: *opus* B f | *ostenditur* ACf: *hostenditur* B

Among the Greeks, one must first refer to Dioscorides' book [...]. But his book that exists in Latin translation from the ancient period is different from our first exemplar. Indeed this one [the first exemplar] is organized through the alphabetical order in Latin whereas that one [the ancient translation] is structured in five books, as it can be demonstrated from its Prologue itself. Moreover, many chapters are lacking in this one [the first exemplar] but are preserved in that one [the ancient translation]. There are even some additions in this book [the first exemplar] that are not from this author: it can be established thanks to Serapion's *De simplicibus* and thanks to that book [the ancient translation].

Simon makes the distinction between two forms of Dioscorides in Latin:
- An ancient Latin translation, organized in five books with a prologue, exactly like the original Greek treatise.
- A Latin *Alphabetical Dioscorides*, which omits numerous chapters and contains apocryphal additions.

To determine what is or is not authentic, Simon refers to the quotations of Dioscorides in the *Liber Serapionis de simplicibus medicinis*:[5] what does not appear there is suspected to be unauthentic.

We can now compare this statement with what we know about the Latin manuscript tradition of Dioscorides.[6] There have been at least three Latin translations of *De materia medica* before the Renaissance: they are called translations A, B, and C. Translations A and B are not directly preserved: we know them only through quotations within other texts and authors. For example, Translation A is mainly preserved in a treatise known as *De herbis femininis*.[7] Only the most recent (Translation C) has come directly to us, through several manuscripts: it should be dated to the sixth century and it has been edited in modern times.[8] It is often referred to as 'Dioscorides Longobardus', the name of its most famous manuscripts (München, *BSB Clm* 337, of the tenth century).[9] But during the Middle Ages, this translation was not widely known.

---

5 As it has recently been demonstrated, this is a Latin translation of the Arabic treatise called Kitāb al-Adwiya al-mufrada (*Book on simple drugs*) by Ibn Wāfid, a pharmacologist living in Toledo in the eleventh century, which relies mainly on Dioscorides and Galen, see: Peter Dilg, "The Liber aggregatus in medicinis simplicibus of Pseudo-Serapion: An influential work of medical Arabism," in Charles Burnett and Anna Contadini (Eds.), *Islam and the Italian Renaissance*, Warburg Institute Colloquia 5 (London: The Warburg Institute, 1999), 221–231 and Peter E. Pormann, 'Yūḥannā ibn Sarābiyūn: Further Studies into the Transmission of his Works", in *Arabic sciences and philosophy* 14 (2004): 236-238. The Latin *De simplicibus medicinis* was first edited in 1473 with the attribution of the translation to Simon himself and to the Jew Abraham of Tortuso (actually this last must be the only translator): *Liber Serapionis agregatus in medicinis simplicibus, translatio Symonis Januensis, interprete Abraam Judaeo tortuosiensi, de arabico in latinum*, (Milano: Antonio Zarotto, 1473).

6 This point has been very accurately studied by Arsenio Ferraces Rodríguez, whose conclusions I will only sum up here. See for example: Arsenio Ferraces Rodríguez, *Fito-zooterapia antigua y altomedieval: textos y doctrinas* (A Coruña: Univ. da Coruña, Servizo de Publicacións, 1999).

7 Edition: Heinrich F. Kästner (ed.), "Pseudo-Dioscoridis *De herbis femininis, Hermes*, 31 (1896), 578-636, with an *addendum* in *Hermes*, 32 (1897), 160. A. Ferraces Rodríguez is preparing a new edition of it, hopefully to be soon published.

8 Edition: Konrad Hofmann, T.M. Auracher, "Der Longobardische Dioskorides des Marcellus Virgilius", *Romanische Forschungen*, 1, (1883), 49-105, Book I with prologue; Theordor M. Auracher, Hermann Stadler, "Die Berner Fragmente des lateinischen Dioskorides", *Archiv für lateinische Lexicographie und Grammatik*, 10 (1898): 117-124, only some fragments; Hermann Stadler, "Dioscorides Longobardus (Cod. Lat. Monac. 337)", *Romanische Forschungen* 10 (1899): 181-247, 369-446, book II and III; Hermann Stadler, "Dioscorides Longobardus (Cod. Lat. Monac. 337)", *Romanische Forschungen*, 11 (1901): 1-93, 94-121, book IV and variants of codex Paris, *BNF lat.* 9332 for book II and III; Hermann Stadler, "Dioscorides Longobardus (Cod. Lat. Monac. 337)", *Romanische Forschungen*, 13 (1902): 161-243, book V; Hermann Stadler, "Dioscorides Longobardus (Cod. Lat. Monac. 337)", *Romanische Forschungen*,14 (1903): 601-637, index; Hermann Stadler," Die Vorrede des lateinischen Dioskorides", *Archiv für lateinische Lexikographie und Grammatik*, 12 (1902), 11-20, prologue. Book I has been re-edited (but without the prologue) by: Haralambie Mihăescu, *Dioscoride latino materia medica libro primo* (Iasi: Terek, 1938). On these editions, see: Bengt Löfstedt, "Textkritische Notizen zu Dioscurides Latinus", *Romanobarbarica* 18 (2003-2005): 91-95.

9 Photographs of this manuscript can be found in the digital library of the BSB: http://www.digitale-sammlungen.de

Indeed, in the last centuries of the Middle Ages, Dioscorides was most frequently transmitted in Latin as an alphabetical re-elaboration, the origin of which is still not known with certainty. The main source of this Latin *Alphabetical Dioscorides* was Translation C but many other fonts were used, among which (as I have recently tried to show), was an exemplary of Translation B.[10] This Latin *Alphabetical Dioscorides* had a very wide diffusion at the end of the Middle Ages. Unfortunately, it was not edited in modern time and we have to refer to Renaissance editions.[11]

Now, if we come back to Simon, we will notice that this statement about the manuscript tradition exactly fits what Simons says and, furthermore, what we can conclude from the analysis of Simon's work. It is indeed possible to prove that Simon directly read one manuscript of each of these two forms of Dioscorides in Latin. After having analysed, not all, but a large number of Dioscorides' quotations in the *Clavis sanationis*, I can say that:

- Simon's main source, what he calls 'Dyascorides' without any more precision, what is his '*primum exemplar*', first exemplar, is the alphabetical re-elaboration. It was very convenient for him, because it was alphabetical, exactly like the *Clavis sanationis*.
- The secondary source is what he calls '*antiqua translatio*', the ancient translation: this is a manuscript of Translation C. He generally refers to this as '*in uero Dyascoride*', in the true Dioscorides.

In practical terms, the distinction is quite difficult for us to make, because the *Alphabetical Dioscorides* mainly quotes Translation C. However, through details, we note that when the two versions are very close (as happens in most cases), Simon prefers to quote the alphabetical Dioscorides, probably because it is more accurate in a grammatical point of view whereas Translation C is written in a quite 'vulgar' Latin.[12] As an illustration of this fact, we can compare the four texts of the chapter dedicated to the thistle:

---

10 Marie Cronier, "Le Dioscoride alphabétique latin et les traductions latines du *De materia medica.*" in Brigitte Maire, David Langslow (Eds.), *Body, Disease and Treatment in a Changing World. Latin texts and contexts in ancient and medieval medicine.* Proceedings of the IX International Conference "Ancient Latin Medical Texts.' Hulme Hall, University of Manchester, 5th-8th September 2007. (Lausanne: BHMS, 2010), 189-200.

11 *Dioscorides de materia medica a Petro Paduano traductus, Colle per Johannem Allemanum de Medemblick*, 1478 (reeditions: Lyon 1512, Venezia 1514).

12 A very accurate linguistic analysis of translation–C can be read in: Haralambie Mihăescu, "La versione latina di Dioscoride, tradizione manoscritta, critica del testo, cenno linguistico." *Ephemeris Dacoromana* 8 (1938): 298-348.

Greek original	Translation-C [13]	Alphabetical Dioscorides (letter C, chap. 17)	Simon, *Clauis sanationis*
Κρίσσιον· ἁπαλὸν καυλίον ἐστίν, ὡς δίπηχυ, τρίγωνον τὸ κάτωθεν, ἀκάνθιά τε ἐκ διαστήματος ἐπ' αὐτῷ μαλακά· τὰ δὲ φύλλα βουγλώσσῳ ἐμφερῆ, δασέα μετρίως καὶ μικρότερα, ὑπόλευκα, ἀκανθώδη τοῖς πέρασι· τὸ δὲ ἀνωτάτω τοῦ καυλοῦ περιφερές, δασύ, καὶ ἐπ' αὐτοῦ κεφάλια ἀκροπόρφυρα, ἐκπαππούμενα.[14]	Crisio: Virga est mollis, longa duobus cubitis, trium angulorum, et spinosa est, circa qua folia sunt mollia, similia buglossu, sed aspriora et minora et subalba et spinosa; quae uirga in capite rotunda est et aspera; super qua capitella sunt purpurea, in quibus uelut cani sebu apparent.	Crision: Virga est mollis *et* longa duobus cubitis, trium angulorum, et spinosa est *cum tirsulis purpureis atque senescentibus,* circa quos folia sunt mollia et similia buglosso, sed asperiora et minora et subalbida et spinosa; que uirga in capite est rotunda. et aspera, super quam capitella sunt purpurea, in quibus uelut *canapi semen apparet.*	Crision . Dya. 'Virga est mollis *et* longa duobus cubitis, trium angulorum, spinosa *cum tirsulis purpureis atque senescentibus,* circa quos folia sunt mollia similia buglose, sed asperiora et minora, subalbida et spinosa; que uirga in capite rotunda est et aspera, supra quam capitella sunt purpurea in quibus ueluti *canapis semen apparet.'*

(*Apparatus ad Simonem : mollis* AC : *molis* B | *tirsulis* AC: *tyrsulis* B | *mollia* AC: *molia* B | *buglosse* A: *buglose* BC | *subalbida et spinosa* B: om. AC | *capitella* AC: *capitela* B | *canapis* AC: *canapi* B)

We can note that the three versions are very close but that Simon and the *Alphabetical Dioscorides* share some minor variants, for example an addition ('*cum tirsulis purpureis atque senescentibus*', with little purple and white [like the hair of old people] stems) coming from another translation and being most probably a variant for the last words (κεφάλια ἀκροπόρφυρα, ἐκπαππούμενα, *purple-tipped heads that become plumed*, only transmitted through an altered form '*uelut(i) canapi(s) semen apparet*', it appears like the seed of '*canapi*', among Simon and the *Alphabetical Dioscorides*) inserted at a wrong place.

---

13 Edition: Stadler, Dioscorides Longobardus, 1901, 56: IV, 114 de crisio.

14 Cf. ed. Wellmann, IV, 118 (κρίσσιον/*krission*): The thistle: it is a tender little stalk, about two cubits tall, triangular at its lower part, having on it at intervals soft little thorns. The leaves are like those of bugloss, moderately rough and smaller, whitish, and prickly at the ends; but the topmost part of the stalk is round, rough, and on it there are purple-tipped heads that become plumed.

In fact, Simon quotes Translation C only when both versions differ significantly; for example in the chapter dedicated to 'pelicinus' (axe weed), where Simon first quotes 'Dyascorides':[15]

Pelicinus. Dya<scorides>: '*Nascitur in triticea segete et ordeacea, cum laminis siue fibris semine plenis, amaris, flauis, baccis* [= axi?] *similibus, nascitur in plurimis et tenuibus ramis. Folia habet pussilla et granula in foliculis sunt trina subruffa et amara ualde. miscetur in antidotis et cetera'.*
2 *baccis* AC : *bacis* B | *plurimis* AC : *pulueris* B |
3 *folia* AB : *follia* C | *pussilla* A: *pusila* B *pussilia* C
4 *miscetur* AC : *miscentur* B
The axe weed. Dioscorides: 'It grows in wheat and barley fields, with pods or lobes which are full of seed, with a bitter taste, red, similar to berry [axe].[16] It grows in numerous and tender branches. It has small leaves and its seeds, in pods, are in groups of three, pale-red, and very bitter. It is used for preparing antidotes, etc.'

This is exactly the text of the *Alphabetical Dioscorides*,[17] which is very different from the equivalent in Translation C. This explains why Simon then adds another chapter, bearing almost the same title:

Pelecinus. In vero Dyas<coride>. '*Herba est habens folia similia ciceris, folliculos similes silique grece, ubi et semen est. ipsum uelut assindi duo rostra habens, unde et pelecinos dicta est quod assi pelix dicta est. gustu amagra, nascitur uero infra in triticum aut ordeum'.*
1 *pelecinus* AC: *pelecius* B | *habens folia* AC: *folia habens* B | *folliculos* AC: *foliculos* B
2 *est ipsum* AC: *ipsum est* B | *uelut* AC: *uelud* B | *assindi* AC : *assia* B |
3 *pelecinos* AC: *pelicinos* B | *assi* AC: *asi* B | *amagra* A: *amara* B, *amaga* C | *in* AC: om. B

The axe weed. In the true Dioscorides: 'It is an herb that has leaves similar to those of chickpea, and pods similar to those of the carob, in which is the seed. The seed itself is like an 'axe' with two 'heads'. Hence it is also called '*pelecinos'*, because the axe is called '*pelix'* [in Greek]. It has a bitter taste. It grows among wheat or barley.'

---

15 Cf. ed. Wellmann III, 130 (ἡδύσαρον/hēdysaron): ἡδύσαρον τὸ ὑπὸ τῶν μυρεψῶν καλούμενον πελεκῖνος· θάμνος ἐστὶ φυλλάρια ἔχων ἐρεβίνθῳ ὅμοια, λοβοὺς δὲ κερατίοις ἐοικότας, ἐν οἷς τὸ σπέρμα πυρρόν, ὅμοιον πελέκει ἀμφιστόμῳ, ὅθεν καὶ ὠνόμασται, πικρὸν γευσαμένῳ, εὐστόμαχον ποθέν· μείγνυται δὲ καὶ ἀντιδότοις (...) φύεται δὲ ἐν κριθαῖς καὶ πυροῖς. The axe weed which unguent makers call *pelecinos*: it is shrub having little leaves like the leaves of the chickpea and pods resembling little horns, wherein lies red seed, similar to a two-edged battleaxe, whence it was named. It tastes bitter and it is wholesome when drunk. They mix it with antidotes (...) It grows among barley and wheat.
16 '*Baccis'* (berries) is most probably a correction (and *lectio facilior*) for '*accis'*, that is 'axis' or '*assis'* (axe).
17 Ed. 1478, letter P, chap. nr. 46.

This last text is exactly that of Translation C:[18] we can notice that Simon considers it as more authentic than the first chapter attributed to Dioscorides and coming from the alphabetical version.

The second case when Simon quotes the 'ancient translation' is when the chapter is omitted in the *Alphabetical Dioscorides*. This is for example the case of the entry dedicated to the plant called *onoma* (stone bugloss):[19]

Onoma. Dya<scorides>: 'Aut nomidana aut flonitin aut nomen dixerunt, folia habet similia anchuse, sed oblonga et molliora, unius palmi habens altitudinem, spansa super terram sicut ancusa, sed nec astam habet nec semen nec florem, radix est illi tenera et minus fortis et rufa, nascitur locis asperis et cetera'.
1 *flonitin* AC *flontin* B | *nomen* AC: *nomi* B
2 *anchuse* AC: *ancuse* B | *oblonga* AC: *oblunga* B | *spansa* AC: *spansam* B
3 *sed* AC: om. B | *nec semen nec florem* AC: *nec florem nec semen* B
4 *rufa* AC: *ruffa* B
Onoma. Dioscorides: 'It is also called *nomidana*, or *flonitin*, or *nomen*. It has leaves similar to those of the alkanet but oblong and softer. It is one palm high and spread on the ground like the alkanet but it has neither stem nor seed nor flower. Its root is thin, with no strength, and red. It grows in rocky places'.

Although Simon does not introduce it with the precision '*in uero Dyascoride*', in the true Dioscorides, this chapter obviously comes from Translation C, in which the equivalent is almost identical: this occurs because this chapter is totally omitted in the Latin *Alphabetical Dioscorides*.

Nevertheless, to sum up, we can affirm that when he quotes Translation C, Simon almost always (but with some exceptions) uses the precision '*in uero Dyascoride*', in the true Dioscorides, whereas when he only says 'D.', or 'Dya.', or nothing, he generally quotes the *Alphabetical Dioscorides*.

We now have to examine the question of which exact manuscript he read; which is very difficult to establish. Concerning the *Alphabetical Dioscorides*, it seems impossible to determine which he read, since there exist no modern critical edition, nor any complete study of its manuscript tradition[20] at the moment. We must confess that for Translation C, it is quite difficult too. It has been said that Simon's exemplar was more complete than the manuscript used for the edition of Translation C (codex

---

18 Edition: Stadler, Dioscorides Longobardus, 1899, 434: book III, chap. 141, *De pelecino*.
19 Ed Wellmann III, 131 (ὄνοσμα/*onosma*).
20 Riddle, John M. "The Latin Alphabetical Dioscorides Manuscript Group". In Proceedings of the XIIIth International Congress for the History of Science (Moscow 1971). Moscow: Nauka, 1974, Section IV, 204-209. Reprint: Riddle, John M. *Quid pro quo. Studies in the history of drugs*. Aldershot: Variorum, 1992, section V.

Monacensis Clm 337)[21] but until now I have not been able to verify this assertion. I can only say that I have noticed that Simon's manuscript generally bears the same *lacunae*, as do the manuscripts we know today. For example, the beginning of the chapter dealing with tamarisk,[22] Simon has to quote through the quotations of Dioscorides transmitted in pseudo-Serapion's *Liber de simplicibus* (see *infra*). Moreover, Simon never does mention any illustrations in the ancient translation; though this is not surprising, since among our manuscripts, only one has illustrations (the codex *Monacensis Clm* 337), whereas all the others do not.

3. Another Testimony of Latin Dioscorides for Simon: *De herbis femininis*

As I have mentioned above, this is a small treatise, dealing with seventy-one plants, of which about sixty percent come from another translation of Dioscorides (Translation A)[23], and was widely known during the Middle Ages. In these conditions, it is not surprising to notice that Simon had access to it and made use of it in *Clavis sanationis*. In fact, he does not expressly attribute it to Dioscorides but (as far as I have seen) he always quotes it after having mentioned Dioscorides. This treatise is described by Simon in different ways: for example '*in libro antiquo*', in the ancient book; '*liber antiquus hystoriatus*', the ancient illustrated book; or '*secundum descriptionem (...) alterius cuiusdam antiqui libri ubi herbe errant depicte*', according to the description... of a second ancient book where the herbs were pictured. I have listed at least five quotations but there may be more. Here is just one example:

> *Sion. Liber antiquus ystoriacus: 'Est que a Latinis labes appellatur, alii † auri uiridem † dicunt, nascitur locis aquosis. Folia eius olixatro* [= *olusatro*] *similia, minora tamen et gustu aromatica'.*
>
> 1 *labes* AC: *laber* B
>
> 3 *gustu* AC: *gusta* B

---

21 Agostino Paravicini Bagliani, "Le biblioteche curiali duecentesche." in: *Libri, lettori e biblioteche dell'Italia medievale (secoli IX-XV). Fonti, testi, utilizzazione del libro*, ed. Giuseppe Lombardi and Donatella Nebbiai Dalla Guarda, (Roma: ICCU, (2000), 271.

22 Greek text in ed. Wellmann I, 87 (μυρική/*myrikē*); Latin text of translation-C in Mihăescu, *Dioscoride latino...*, 50.

23 The relations between *De herbis femininis* (sometime also called *De herbis feminis* or *Ex herbis feminis*) and translation-A have been established and very precisely analyzed by Ferraces Rodríguez, *Estudios sobre textos latinos...*. On this treatise, see also: John Riddle, "'Pseudo-Dioscorides' 'Ex herbis feminis' and Early Medieval Medical Botany." *Journal of the History of Biology* 14 (1981): 43-81.

Water parsnip. In the ancient illustrated book: 'It is the plant that Latins call labes, but some others call it [*laurum uiridem*, green laurel].[24] It grows in water. Its leaves are similar to Alexanders but smaller, and they have an aromatic taste.'

This exactly corresponds to chapter sixty-nine of *De herbis femininis*,[25] which comes from Translation A of Dioscorides' *De materia medica*.[26]

However, one has to stay careful, since the words '*liber antiquus ubi herbe erant depicte*' the ancient book where the herbs were pictured, in Simon's *Clavis sanationis* can also designate other treatises: pseudo-Apuleius' *Herbarius,* for example.[27]

4. Dioscorides in Greek

It is often said that Simon did not have great knowledge of Greek language, although he often explains the names of the plants through etymology of Greek roots.[28] Indeed, he never quotes the Greek text of Dioscorides. However, he sometimes refers to some illustrations he says he has seen 'in Greek manuscripts' but, until now, I have noticed only one passage where he says this Greek illustrated manuscript is by Dioscorides:

Lagopos. Grece est dictu pes leporis. Dya<scorides> : 'Dicta est a similitudine leporini pedis, nascitur in pratis et locis cultis et ubi oliue habundant et cetera.' Hanc ego uidi depictam in libro greco Dy<ascoridis> habentem folia pusilla, triangulate forme, per omnes ramulos utrinque ab ambobus lateribus contiguata,

---

24 These words are already corrupt in the source, *De herbis femininis*: *aurum uiride* ed. Kästner. In personal communication, resulting from unpublished investigation, Arsenio Ferraces Rodríguez proposes the emendation: *laurum uiridem* (green laurel), which seems very satisfying. However, when editing Simon's text, we have to keep the corrupted version as it was in the quoted source.

25 Edition: Kästner, "Addendum", 160; Greek original: ed Wellmann II, 127 (σίον/*sion*).

26 The others four entries where *De herbis femininis* is quoted are: 1) Achantis leuce (= excerpt from chap. 1: ed. Kastner 591, l. 7); 2) *Achantos* (= chap. 3, *acantum*, ed. p. 592); 3) *Licanis stiphaica* (= chap. 68, *lichnis*: ed. p. 635); 4) *Splenion et asplenon et scolopendriam* (= chap. 40, *splenios*, ed. p. 616).

27 This is for example the case of the entry *artemisia* where, under the expression '*Quodam libro antiquo ubi herbe erant depicte*', in some ancient book where the herbs where illustrated, Simon obviously refers to chap. 10-12 of the *Herbarius* of pseudo-Apuleius, edition: Ernestus Howald and Henricus E. Sigerist, *Antonii Musae de herba uettonica liber. Pseudoapulei herbarius. Anonymi de taxone liber. Sexti Placiti medicinae ex animalibus, etc.*, Corpus Medicorum Latinorum (Leipzig and Berlin: Teubner, 1927), 42-45.

28 For example: Danielle Jacquart, "La coexistence du grec et de l'arabe dans le vocabulaire médical du latin médiéval: l'effort linguistique de Simon de Gênes." in Michèle Groult (Ed.), *Transferts de vocabulaire dans les sciences*, (Paris: CNRS, 1988), 277-290.

per totum humilem plantulam expansam super faciem terre, in multis locis nascitur (...).[29]

1 *Dia.* B: *om.* AC | *similitudine* AB: *simimilitudine* C

2 *leporini pedis* AC: *pedis leporine* B

3 *Hanc ego uidi* AC: *ego uidi hanc* B

Hare's foot trefoil. In Greek it is called hare's foot. Dioscorides: 'It has such name because it resembles the foot of the hare. It grows in the meadows and the cultivated fields, and where the olives are abundant, etc.' I personally saw it pictured in a Greek book by Dioscorides: it had small leaves in a triangular form, being situated together in both sides of each branch; it is in general a very small plant that spreads over the ground. It grows in many places.

The fact that Simon here proposes his own description, made from the illustrations he sees, is quite rare in the *Clavis sanationis* but can be explained by the basic quality of Dioscorides' description. This brings up the question of the availability for Simon of Greek illustrated Dioscorides manuscripts. To my knowledge, there were only two such manuscripts in Western Europe (more precisely: in Italy) at the end of the thirteenth century:

- *Parisinus gr.* 2179: copied in the Syro-palestinian region at the end of the eighth century but brought to Southern Italy (Terra d'Otranto) before the middle of the thirteenth century (because it was copied there at that time into two Greek apographs). It bears several notes by thirteenth- and fourteenth-century Latin hands, but as far as I know, it remained in a monastery in Terra d'Otranto until the sixteenth century.[30]

- *Neapolitanus gr.* 1* (*olim Vindobonensis suppl. gr.* 28): copied in Italy probably in the seventh century, it seems to have remained first in Calabria then in the Naples region, most probably in a monastery, until the eighteenth century. It also bears annotations by Latin hands of the thirteenth- and fourteenth-centuries, mainly next to the figures of the plants (the illustrations being the major interest of this manuscript for the Latin annotators). (online facsimile: http://www.wdl.org/en/item/10690/)

We do not have enough knowledge about Simon's biography to say whether it is possible or not that Simon had travelled to such monasteries and got access to these manuscripts, but what I can say is that the description of the illustrations

---

[29] Greek original chapter: ed. Wellmann IV, 17 (λαγώπουν/*lagōpoun*): although the name of Dioscorides is lacking in some testimonies of Simon's tradition, the sentence at the beginning of this entry comes from the equivalent chapter in the alphabetical Latin Dioscorides (itself coming from Translation C with minor changes).

[30] This information comes from my personal research, which has been included in my PhD thesis: Marie Cronier, *Recherches sur l'histoire du texte du* De materia medica *de Dioscoride,* (Diss. École pratique des Hautes Études, Paris, 2007), 83-95. See online facsimile of the manuscript in http://gallica.bnf.fr.

he gives does not fit the illustrations of these two Dioscorides manuscripts. In the Naples manuscript (f.92r), the leaves are not triangular and the plant is not creeping, whereas in the Paris manuscript (f. 77r), the leaves are a little more triangular but the plant is not creeping.

However, there may be a quite simple explanation of this phenomenon. Since the beginning of the chapter comes from Dioscorides, but in some testimonies does not bear the mention of this author's name, we are allowed to suspect that the mention 'Dya.' that appears after 'in libro greco', in the Greek book, may have been slightly displaced and was originally to be written not here but at the beginning of the entry. In a consequence, Simon would only speak about 'a Greek manuscript', not necessarily by Dioscorides, and there would not be any more mention of a Greek illustrated Dioscorides in the *Clavis sanationis*.

Indeed, there are three other cases where Simon speaks about some pictures he has seen in Greek manuscripts, without saying expressly they are Dioscorides manuscripts: in the chapters dedicated to the bear's-foot,[31] the miltwaste (in two different entries),[32] and the hackberry.[33] These illustrated Greek books do not seem to be by Dioscorides. In any case, what Simon tells us about their pictures does not fit the illustrations that have been preserved for the corresponding chapters by

---

31 *Achantos seu achantinos* (...) *Reperii in libro greco hystoriato herbam depictam ut hic describitur, flore albo, pederos uocatam* (...). *Achantos* [Bear's-foot] or *Achantinos.* I found in a Greek illustrated book this plant with a picture like it is described here, with a white flower, and called *pederos.* The original Greek chapter by Dioscorides is ed. Wellmann III, 17 (ἄκανθος/*akanthos*).

32 This discussion appears in two chapters, bearing similar titles and corresponding to one original Greek chapter (ed. Wellmann III, 134: ἄσπληνος/*asplēnos*): *asplenon* and *splenion* or *scolopendria.* The question is to determine whether they are dealing with the same plant and whether this plant is 'lingua ceruina' (deer's-tongue) or 'ceterach'. Simon tries to find arguments from the illustrations but he is forced to conclude that there is a general confusion even among the pictures in the manuscripts. This problem seems to have been of interest during the Middle Ages, as can be attested for example in the Naples Dioscorides manuscript where (f. 134r) Latin hands of the thirteenth - fourteenth centuries have written the names *ceterac* et *scholopendrion* next to the figure of σκολοπένδριον/*skolopendrion* (itself being associated to the text of <ἄσπληνος/*asplēnos*>!). It would deserve a wider discussion, which can not take place here.

33 *Lothos arbor* (...) *In libro uero greco ubi depicte sunt herbe et arbores est illa quam fabam grecam ydiomate nostro uocamus.* Hackberry ['lotos'-tree] ... But in the Greek book where the herbs and the trees are illustrated, it is the tree that in our language we call 'faba greca' [Greek bean]. This corresponds to one of the (numerous) chapters called λωτός / *lōtos* in *De materia medica*, hence the discussion to determine which plant is dealt with (here: ed. Wellmann I, 117: λωτὸς τὸ δένδρον / *lōtos to dendron*, the 'lotos-tree'). To my knowledge, only two Greek Dioscorides manuscripts bear illustration for it (the Greek manuscripts containing illustrations for trees being in general very rare): New York, Morgan Library, M. 652, of the beginning of the tenth century (f. 256v), but this is a Constantinopolitan manuscript that reached the Occident not before the end of the 18th century; and Mount Athos, Monastery Megistis Lavras, codex Ω 75, of the eleventh century (f. 174v), a manuscript also produced in Constantinople and that never came to Occidental Europe.

Dioscorides in Greek manuscripts. However, I must confess I cannot say precisely which kind of manuscript Simon is talking about: it could have been an anonymous herbal that has not come down to us. Whereas many Latin illustrated herbals have been transmitted to us, the situation is very different for the Byzantine evidence, of which the number of books bearing botanical illustration is quite small.

In any case, we can sum up the situation by saying that there is very little evidence that Simon has used a Greek Dioscorides manuscript. However, he quite probably had access to some Greek illustrated manuscripts, which were not by Dioscorides but may be some popular and anonymous illustrated herbals.

5. Dioscorides in Arabic

There are two scenarios. Firstly: Simon's quotations of Dioscorides according to pseudo-Serapion. As I have said above, Simon sometimes resorts to 'Serapion' to determine if a chapter attributed to Dioscorides is authentic or not. Moreover, when Translation C and the *Alphabetical Dioscorides* are incomplete, Simon can quote Dioscorides' words according to Serapion. I will give just one example of this phenomenon, which is not frequent, in the chapter dedicated to the tamarisk:

> *Tamariscus. Quamuis in antiqua translatione Dy<ascoridis> inueniatur ca<pitulum> de tamarisco et uocatur murice; non est tamen capitulum Dya<scoridis> secundum quod apparet in Ser<apionis> li<bro> in quo sic ex uerbo Dya<scoridis>: 'Est, inquit, arbor erecta que nascitur in aquis, intelligo iuxta aquas uel locis aquosis, habet fructum qui assimilatur floribus (...).'*[34]
> 3 *in Ser. li.* AC : *in libro Serap.* B |
> 4 *arbor erecta* AC: *errecta arbor* B |
> Tamarisk. Although in the ancient translation of Dioscorides there is a chapter about tamarisk, that is called 'murice', it is not the Dioscorides chapter according to what appears in Serapion's book, in which there is this quotation attributed to Dioscorides: 'He says this is a tall tree that grows in waters, I understand next to the waters or in humid places; it has a fruit that is similar to the flowers...'

Simon is annoyed by the fact that his two Latin Dioscorides translations, which are here almost identical, do not contain any physical description of this tree but only mention its therapeutic properties (which, as we have seen, Simon is not

---

[34] These words exactly correspond to the beginning of the chapter called '*tamariscus*' in the 1473 edition of pseudo-Serapion's *De simplici medicina* (f. 27v). Original Greek chapter: ed. Wellmann I, 87(μυρικὴ/ *myrike*).

interested in with regards to *De materia medica*). However, he has noticed that in the chapter dedicated to the same plant (*tamariscus*), pseudo-Serapion quotes explicitly Dioscorides, giving a description of it. In fact, both pseudo-Serapion's quotation and that of the two Latin versions come from the same original Greek chapter by Dioscorides but, for an undetermined reason, Translation C (followed by the *Alphabetical Dioscorides*) omits the first part of this chapter (with the description). The words quoted by Simon fit the original Greek but differ from the three already known Latin translations: this proves that they come from a translation from Arabic into Latin, actually that of Ibn Wāfid 's *Book on simple drugs*, itself quoting Dioscorides through an Arabic translation from Greek.

The second case – even more rare than the previous one – is when Simon says that he is quoting directly from an Arabic Dioscorides manuscript. Let's examine one example of it, in the chapter dedicated to the feverfew (Pyrethrum parthenium):

> *Achauĕ. (...) Item in Dya<scoride> arabico libro primo: 'Senchaet amaracinum est dehen alachauĕ, id est oleum de achauĕ, et cetera'. Item idem in libro .iii.: 'Barthenion, ('b' ponens pro 'p' littera qua carent Arabes): Sunt inquit qui uocant eam amaracum et ipsa est alachauĕ'.*
>
> 1 *in Dya. arabico* AC: *Dia. in arabico* B | *senchaet* AC: *seuhaet* B | *amaracinum* AC: *amaracum* B
>
> 2 *idem* AC: *ibidem* B | *barthenion: barthemon* ABC
>
> 4 *alachauĕ* AC: *alachanĕ* B
>
> Feverfew ... Then, in the Arabic Dioscorides, book one: '*Senchaet* of feverfew is dehen al-achauĕ, that is to say: achauĕ oil, et cetera.' Then in book tree, the same: '*Barthenion* (using 'b' instead of 'p', a letter that lacks in Arabic): Some people, he says, call it *amaracum*, and this is alachavĕ [the feverfew].'[35]

Indeed, we can find back in the Arabic translation of Dioscorides[36] the very Arabic words Simon is quoting. First, in Book I of this translation

---

35 Original Greek chapter: ed. Wellmann III, 138 (παρθένιον/parthenion).

36 Although we considered until recently that there have existed three Arabic translations of Dioscorides, Manfred Ullmann has discovered a fourth one, probably more ancient than the three others and attested only in the manuscript of Istanbul, Süleymaniye Kütüphanesi, Ayasofia 3704: see Manfred Üllmann, *Untersuchungen zur arabischen Überlieferung der Materia medica des Dioskurides.* (Wiesbaden: Harrassowitz 2009). However, only one of them has been published: César Emil Dubler, *La "Materia médica' de Dioscórides. Transmisión medieval y renacentista*, (Barcelona, Tipografia Emporium, 1952-1959), 6 vol., vol. 2: *La versión árabe de la 'Materia médica' de Dioscórides. Texto, variantes e índices.* Its author was Iṣṭifān ibn Basīl (Stephen, the son of Basil), a disciple of the famous translator Ḥunain ibn Isḥāq, living in Bagdad in the middle of the ninth century. This translation was the most wide known in the Arabic world during the Middle Ages. I have made a comparison only with Stephen's translation, and thus noticed that Simon's words fit it, but a comparison with the three others translations may be of interest.

(as well as in the original Greek treatise), the chapter dealing with the unguent of *amarakon* begins this way: صنعة اماراقينن و هو دهن الاقحوان (ṣanʿatu āmārāqīnuni wa huwa duhnun al-uqhuwāni, recipe of *amaraqinun*, that is unguent of feverfew).[37] Then, in Book III, here is the beginning of the chapter on feverfew: فرثانيون و هو الاقحوان. و من الناس من يسمه اماراقن (farṯāniyūnun, wa huwa al-uqhuwānun, wa min an-nāsi man yusmiha āmārāqunun, *Farthenion*. This is the feverfew. Some people call it *amaraqun*)[38]. Simon transcribes the Arabic words in a quite accurate way, although of course, not corresponding to the actual scientific criteria. For example, he transcribes لاقحوان *al-uqhuwān* through 'alachauē', صنعة ṣanʿat through *senchaet* and دهن *duhn* through *dehen*. We can thus imagine that he had direct access to an Arabic Dioscorides manuscript and not only to Latin quotations through Avicenna and pseudo-Serapion. He also may have been able, if not to perfectly read and understand it, at least to decipher some few words, maybe with the help of someone else. In this specific case, however, I must say that all the Arabic Dioscorides manuscripts I know, do transcribe the Greek παρθένιον/parthenion with the initial ف/f, never with the initial ب/b as Simon says his own manuscript does.[39]

It is important that his Arabic Dioscorides preserved the original structure, that is to say that it contained the chapters about oils and unguents in Book I and the chapter about feverfew in Book III, exactly as in the original Greek form. In addition, it must be stressed that Simon's Arabic manuscript contained illustrations, as we can see in the following chapter, dealing with the madwort:[40]

> *Auricula muris (...) Verum ego uidi ipsam depictam in libro D<ioscoridis> arabico diuersam ab aliis plantis.*
> 1 *arabico* AC: *in ara.* B
> 2 *aliis* AC: *his* B
>
> Madwort ... However, I personally saw it illustrated in an Arabic book of Dioscorides differently from the other plants.

---

37 Cf. ed. Wellmann I, 58 (ἀμαράκινον μύρον/*amarakinon myron*); Dubler I, 54. There is no entry called ἀμάρακον/*amarakon* in *De materia medica*, hence the present confusion between two plants: ἀμάρακον/amarakon usually designates the marjoram (*Origanum majorana L.*), a plant which is called σάμψουχον/*sampsouchon* by Dioscorides (III, 39), but, as indicated by Dioscorides himself, ἀμάρακον/*amarakon* is also used as a synonym for παρθένιον/*parthenion*, the feverfew (*Pyrethrym Parthenium*). The Arabic translator only knows this last meaning.

38 Cf. ed. Wellmann III, 138 (παρθένιον/*parthenion*); Dubler III, 131.

39 However, the codex Ayasofia 3704 (see n. 36) does not give any title for this chapter and the Arabic manuscript Paris, *BNF ar.* 4947, the main testimony of a different translation than that edited by Dubler, here bears a lacuna. Photographs of this manuscript and those of the two other Dioscorides Arabic manuscripts of the BNF (nr. 2849 and 2850) are available on the Gallica digital library: http://gallica.bnf.fr

40 Wellmann II, 183 (μυὸς ὦτα/*myos ōta*).

Once again, we have to face the question of the availability of Arabic manuscripts by Dioscorides to Simon of Genoa and I must confess that, to my knowledge, none of the Arabic Dioscorides manuscripts we know today were available in Western Europe at the time of Simon, except in Spain. For example, the manuscripts of Paris, *BNF ar.* 2850, and of Madrid, *BN* 5006, were copied in Al-Andalus in the twelfth to thirteenth century (only the first of them bearing illustrations). In consequence, Spain would be the most likely place for Simon to get access to such a book, although this field surely needs more investigation.

To conclude, we can sum up the situation in this way:

As concerns the Latin sources of Dioscorides, what was available to Simon perfectly fits what we know about Dioscorides' manuscript tradition. He had access to Translation C (an interesting phenomenon, because it was quite rare at this time), to the *Alphabetical Dioscorides* (a medieval re-elaboration of Translation C with many additions), and to the *De herbis femininis* (indirect testimony of Translation A). He does not seem to know a textual version, which would have been lost for us, so his quotations have little interest for editing the Latin Dioscorides. Nevertheless, Simon has a very interesting critical attitude, which he expresses by comparing both versions and trying to determine what is authentic or not, and, most times, he is right. It is quite remarkable too, that he resorts to indirect Arabic Dioscorides tradition, mainly in the quotations by pseudo-Serapion, so as to determine what is or is not authentic.

Moreover, the study of Simon's quotations of Dioscorides brings up the question of whether he has directly used Greek and Arabic Dioscorides manuscripts. The answer is not easy to establish and has not yet exhaustively been investigated but, for the moment, I would say that his access to Greek Dioscorides is quite problematic whereas he is more likely to have seen Arabic Dioscorides.

Bibliography

Aufmesser, Max. *Etymologische und wortgeschichtliche Erläuterungen zu De materia medica des Pedanius Dioscurides Anazarbeus.* Hildesheim-Zürich-New York: Olms-Weidmann, 2000.

Auracher, Theodor M. and Hermann Stadler. "Die Berner Fragmente des lateinischen Dioskorides." *Archiv für lateinische Lexicographie und Grammatik,* 10 (1898): 117-124.

Cronier, Marie. *Recherches sur l'histoire du texte du* De materia medica *de Dioscoride.* Diss. École pratique des Hautes Études, Paris, 2007.

— "Le Dioscoride alphabétique latin et les traductions latines du De materia medica." In Brigitte Maire and David Langslow (Eds.). *Body, Disease and Treatment in a Changing World. Latin texts and contexts in ancient and medieval medicine. Proceedings of the IX International Conference 'Ancient Latin Medical Texts',* Hulme Hall, University of Manchester, 5th-8th September 2007, 189-200. Lausanne: BHMS, 2010.

Dilg, Peter. "The Liber aggregatus in medicinis simplicibus of Pseudo-Serapion: An influential work of medical Arabism." In Charles Burnett and Anna Contadini (eds.), *Islam and the Italian Renaissance,* Warburg Institute Colloquia 5, 221–231. (London: The Warburg Institute, 1999).

Dioscorides De materia medica, libri quinque, edited by Max Wellmann, 3 vol. Berlin: Weidmann, 1906-1914. Reeditions: Berlin, 2010.

Dioscorides de materia medica a Petro Paduano traductus, Colle per Johannem Allemanum de Medemblick, 1478. Reeditions: Lyon 1512, Venezia 1514.

Dubler, César Émil. *La 'Materia médica' de Dioscórides. Transmisión medieval y renacentista*, 6 vol. Barcelona: Tipografía Emporium, 1952-1959.

Ferraces Rodríguez, Arsenio. *Estudios sobre textos latinos de fitoterapia entre la Antigüedad tardía y la Alta Edad Media*. A Coruña: Universidade da Coruña, Servicio de Publ., 1999.

Hofmann, Konrad, and Theodor M. Auracher. "Der Longobardische Dioskorides des Marcellus Virgilius." *Romanische Forschungen* 1 (1883): 49-105.

Howald, Ernestus, and Henricus E. Sigerist. *Antonii Musae de herba uettonica liber. Pseudoapulei herbarius. Anonymi de taxone liber. Sexti Placiti medicinae ex animalibus, etc.*, Corpus Medicorum Latinorum (Leipzig and Berlin: Teubner, 1927).

Jacquart, Danielle. "La coexistence du grec et de l'arabe dans le vocabulaire médical du latin médiéval : l'effort linguistique de Simon de Gênes." In Martine Groult (Ed.), *Transferts de vocabulaire dans les sciences*. 277- 290. Paris: CNRS, 1988.
Reprint: *La science médicale occidentale entre deux renaissances (XIIe s.-XVe s.).* (Altershot: Variorum, 1997), section X.

Kästner, Heinrich F. "Pseudo-Dioscoridis *De herbis femininis*." *Hermes* 31 (1896): 578.

Kästner, Heinrich F. "Addendum. Pseudo-Dioscoridis *De herbis femininis*." *Hermes* 32 (1897): 160.

Liber Serapionis agregatus in medicinis simplicibus, translatio Symonis Januensis, interprete Abraam Judaeo tortuosiensi, de arabico in latinum (Milano: Antonio Zarotto, 1473).

Löfstedt, Bengt. "Textkritische Notizen zu Dioscurides Latinus." *Romanobarbarica* 18 (2003-2005): 91-95.

Mihăescu, Haralambie. *Dioscoride latino materia medica libro primo*. Iasi: Terek, 1938.

— "La versione latina di Dioscoride, tradizione manoscritta, critica del testo, cenno linguistico." *Ephemeris Dacoroman* 8 (1938): 298-348.

Paravicini-Bagliani, Agostino. "Le biblioteche curiali duecentesche." In: *Libri, lettori e biblioteche dell'Italia medievale (secoli IX-XV). Fonti, testi, utilizzazione del libro*, ed. Giuseppe Lombardi and Donatella Nebbiai Dalla Guarda. 263-275. Roma: ICCU, 2000.

Pedanius Dioscorides of Anazarbus. *De materia medica*, translated by Lily Y. Beck. *Altertumswissenschaftliche Texte und Studien* 38. Hildesheim-Zürich-New York: Olms-Weidmann, 2005.

Pormann, Peter E. "Yūḥannā ibn Sarābiyūn: Further Studies into the Transmission of his Works." *Arabic sciences and philosophy* 14 (2004): 236-238.

Riddle, John M. "The Latin Alphabetical Dioscorides Manuscript Group." In *Proceedings of the XIIIth International Congress for the History of Science* (Moscow 1971). Moscow: Nauka, 1974, Section IV, 204-209. Reprint: Riddle, John M. *Quid pro quo. Studies in the history of drugs*. Aldershot: Variorum, 1992, section V.

— "Pseudo-Dioscorides' '*Ex herbis feminis*' and Early Medieval Medical Botany." *Journal of the History of Biology* 14 (1981): 43-81.

Stadler, Hermann. "Dioscorides Longobardus (Cod. Lat. Monac. 337)." *Romanische Forschungen* 10 (1899): 1-247, 369-446.

— "Dioscorides Longobardus (Cod. Lat. Monac. 337)." *Romanische Forschungen* 11 (1901): 1-93, 94-121.

— "Dioscorides Longobardus (Cod. Lat. Monac. 337)." *Romanische Forschungen* 13 (1902): 161-243.

— "Dioscorides Longobardus (Cod. Lat. Monac. 337)." *Romanische Forschungen* 14 (1903): 601-637.

— "Die Vorrede des lateinischen Dioskorides." *Archiv für lateinische Lexikographie und Grammatik* 12 (1902): 11-20.

Ullmann, Manfred. *Untersuchungen zur arabischen Überlieferung der Materia medica des Dioskurides*. Wiesbaden: Harrassowitz, 2009..

Edited by **Barbara Zipser**

Valerie Knight[1]

Simon and the Tradition of the Latin Alexander of Tralles

Certainly from the late eighth/early ninth century, the Greek *Therapeutica* of the sixth-century Byzantine physician Alexander of Tralles was transmitted in a Latin translation, but with significant additions to, and omissions from, the Greek text. This paper will present evidence from the *Clavis sanationis* that confirms Simon's use of the Latin version and will examine the Latin manuscript tradition of specific entries. It will also briefly consider the glosses attributed to Simon in the 1504 (Lyons) printing, *Practica Alexandri yatros greci cum expositione glose interlinearis Iacobi de Partibus et Ianuensis in margine posite*, edited by Fr. Fradin.

✳

In the preface (Section 4) of the *Clavis sanationis*, Simon tells us that 'after Dioscorides' (*post Diascoridem*) he 'carefully examined' (*diligenter inspexi*) the work of one 'Alexander' (*Alexandri*).

Simon's 'Alexander' is the sixth-century Byzantine physician Alexander of Tralles who, having settled at an unknown date in Rome and following a long career,[2] wrote - in Greek - the *Therapeutica* and *On fevers* (Περὶ πυρετῶν).[3] At some stage, both these works were translated into Latin - certainly by the late eighth/early ninth century, the date of the oldest extant manuscript. David Langslow has called the combination of these two translations the 'Latin Alexander'.[4]

---

1 The author is a (part-time) PhD student at the University of Manchester, funded by the Arts and Humanities Research Council (AHRC).

2 For Alexander's dates and life, see David Langslow, *The Latin Alexander Trallianus: The text and transmission of a Late Latin medical book.* (London: Society for the Promotion of Roman Studies, 2006), 1-4 and notes. I would like to thank David Langslow for allowing me to quote extensively from his book, *The Latin Alexander Trallianus* (2006), and for kindly giving me free access to his electronic transcript of Angers, *Bibl. mun.* 457, as well as for his helpful observations on reading the first draft of this paper. My thanks also to the anonymous reviewers for their invaluable comments. Last, but certainly not least, I thank Barbara Zipser for all her help and encouragement. All errors, oversights and misunderstandings are entirely mine.

3 Alexander also wrote a third work, in the form of a letter, *On intestinal worms* (Περὶ ἐλμίνθων). For a discussion of Alexander's writings, including details of two works ascribed to Alexander that are regarded as spurious (*On eyes* - Περὶ ὀφθαλμῶν - and *On the pulse and urine*), see Langslow *The Latin Alexander Trallianus...*, 4-6 and references therein.

4 *Ibidem*, 5 and n. 33.

Alexander's *Therapeutica* therefore exists in two distinct traditions, one Greek and one Latin.

There are eighteen known manuscripts containing all or part of the Greek *Therapeutica*, ranging in date from the tenth to the seventeenth century,[5] with the first edition printed in 1548. The most recent edition is that of Theodor Puschmann, a doctor himself, published in two volumes in 1878-1879.[6]

There are twenty-one known complete manuscript copies of the Latin Alexander, nineteen of which are extant, ranging in date from the late eighth/early ninth to the sixteenth century.[7] (See Appendix 1 for a full list of these manuscripts, including the *sigla* used by Langslow in his 2006 book *The Latin Alexander Trallianus*).[8] The Latin Alexander was first printed in 1504 at Lyons as the *Practica Alexandri yatros greci*.[9] It is divided into three books: Book 1 contains chapters dealing with hair-loss to pleuritis; Book 2, chapters dealing with coughing to gout; and Book 3, chapters dealing with fevers. (See Appendix 2 for Langslow's stemma, showing the relationship between the manuscripts containing the Latin Alexander and the 1504 Lyons edition.)[10]

Given that Alexander's *Therapeutica* exists in both Greek and Latin, the question arises as to which version did Simon use – or, indeed, did he utilise both? Two statements made by Simon are certainly evidence that he has used the Latin Alexander. The first of these is found in Section 4 of Simon's preface:[11]

---

5 *Ibidem*, 13 and nn. 1-4. For details of these manuscripts and a stemma showing the relationship between them, see Barbara Zipser, "Die *Therapeutica* des Alexander Trallianus: Ein medizinisches Handbuch und seine Überlieferung," in Rosa Maria Piccione and Matthias Perkams (Eds.), *Selecta Colligere, II. Beiträge zur Methodik des Sammelns von Texten in der Spätantike und in Byzanz (Collana Hellenika).* (Alessandria: Edizioni dell'Orso, 2005), 211-234.

6 All references to the Greek *Therapeutica* in this paper are to Theodor Puschmann, *Alexander von Tralles. Original-Text und Übersetzung nebst einer einleitenden Abhandlung. Ein Beitrag zur Geschichte der Medicin*, 2 vols (repr. 1963, Amsterdam: A. M. Hakkert), (Vienna: W. Braumüller, 1878-1879), giving volume (I or II), page and (where appropriate) line number.

7 Langslow, *The Latin Alexander Trallianus...*, 37, notes that '... the manuscript tradition of the Latin Alexander... is one of the richest, if not the richest, known for such an early medieval Latin medical text as the Latin Alexander must be, in particular for such a long text'.

8 *Ibidem*, 37-8; for full details of the individual manuscripts, see also: 40-53.

9 *Practica Alexandri yatros greci cum expositione glose interlinearis Iacobi de partibus et Ianuensis in margine posite*, edited by Fr. Fradin.

10 Reproduced from Langslow, *The Latin Alexander Trallianus...*, Plate XII, with the kind permission of David Langslow.

11 Generally, throughout this paper, where no apparatus existed (at the time of writing) on the *Simon Online* website, I present both the transcription of A (the 1510 printing) taken from the website, alongside my transcription of B (the 1473 printing). Here, I have underlined differences between the two versions.

Preface, § 4 (Transcript A, 1510, last accessed 12.03.12)
Post Dyascoridem Alexandri librum de pratica [sic] *dilligenter* inspexi *qui qui* quamvis tribus *distinguitur* libellis: *tertiuś* qui de febribus est: nec veritatem in *nominibus neque* tanti philosophi seriem videtur *plenius* continere.*

Preface, § 4 (Print B, 1473)
post Diascoridem Alexandri librum de pratica [sic] *diligenter* inspexi *qui* quamvis tribus *distinguatur* libellis *tertius tamen* qui de febribus est nec ueritatem in *omnibus nec* tanti philosophi seriem uidetur *plenarie* continere.*

After Dioscorides I carefully examined the book of Alexander on *pra[c]tica* which although it is divided up in three books, nevertheless the third [book] which is on fevers seems to fully contain neither accuracy in everything nor the context of such a great *philosophus*.

Simon's description of the work being divided into three books, with the third book being on fevers, is a description of the Latin Alexander. As well as the Lyons 1504 edition, all the extant Latin manuscripts, except one, transmit the Latin Alexander in three books, the exception being **P3**: Paris, *BNF lat.* 6882.[12] This is in stark contrast to the Greek tradition, where the division is either into eleven or twelve books.[13]

In the second, found in the latter part of his moderately lengthy entry for *sauich*, Simon explicitly refers to the use of an Alexander 'translated from the Greek':

Sauich (Print B, 1473)[14]
... notandum tamen quod ubicumque habetur in liberis [sic] de arabico translatis sauich apud Dia. et **Alex**. *et Paul(_) et alios* **de greco translatos** *habetur polenta quare secudum [sic] idem uidetur apud grecos uero uocatur alfita ut patet per Gal(_).*

---

12 Langslow, *The Latin Alexander Trallianus...*, 18-19.

13 See Zipser, "Die *Therapeutica* des Alexander Trallianus...", especially p.222. It is worth noting that there is an early thirteenth-century, Spanish or Catalonian, manuscript that transmits the Latin *On fevers* (*De febribus*) independently, a transmission that has no parallel in the Greek tradition (Langslow, *The Latin Alexander Trallianus...*, 5 n. 33, referring to the manuscript Barcelona, *Archivo de la Corona de Aragón, Ripoll* 181; see *ibid.* 90 and 92 for further details and bibliography for this manuscript).

14 Cf. Print A (last accessed 26.10.12): *notandum tamen quod ubicumque habetur in libris* **de greco** [with apparatus: 'de greco ACDQR | de arabico B efgz'] *translatis sauich apud Dya. et Alexan. Paulum et alios de greco translatos habetur polenta quare secundum hoc idem videtur apud grecos vero vocatur alfitis in li. de alimentis. Item Ste. in synonimis dicit quod alfiton est sauich.*

ca. de alfitis in libro de alimentis item Ste. in sinonimis dicit quod alfiton est sauich.
... Note, however, that everywhere it is written in books translated from Arabic [it is] *sauich*; in the writings of Dioscorides and **Alexander** and Paul and others **translated from the Greek**, it is written *polenta*, for which reason we may assume they are synonyms. Among the Greeks, indeed, it is called *alphita*, as is revealed through Galen in the chapter on *alphita* in his book *On foods*. Likewise Stephanus in his *Synonyms* says that *alphita* is *sauich*.

On Dioscorides, see Marie Cronier in this volume. With regard to Paul, Peter Pormann notes that Paul's 'Book III on diseases from tip to toe was translated into Latin in 11th c. south Italy.'[15]

What further evidence is to be found that Simon used the Latin Alexander and is there any evidence at all to suggest that Simon may have used the Greek *Therapeutica*? To explore this question, it is first necessary to consider the differences between the Greek *Therapeutica* and the Latin Alexander.[16] These differences range from what might be thought of as relatively minor discrepancies - from a single word to several sentences[17] - to what can only be considered as major variations in content.

The Latin Alexander contains a considerable number of glosses,[18] which are described by Langslow as:

> ... [the] more elaborate explication, of technical terms and concepts which are employed, usually without explanation,[19] in the Greek original ... Usually, these involve either simply highlighting that the word is Greek ... or providing a Latin gloss or terminological equivalent ... [28] ... usually with an explicit reference to Greek terminology ...[20]

Significant sections found in the Greek *Therapeutica* are missing from the Latin Alexander. In Book 1 of the Latin Alexander some remedies for epilepsy present in the Greek text are missing. In Book 2, a larger number of remedies

---

15 Peter Porman, "Paulos of Aigina (ca 630 – 670 CE?)," in Paul T. Keyser and Georgia L. Irby-Massie (Eds.), *The encyclopedia of ancient natural scientists*. (London and New York, NY: Routledge, 2008), 625.

16 For a comparison of the Greek *Therapeutica* and the Latin version, see Langslow, *The Latin Alexander Trallianus...*, 17–35.

17 Langslow, *The Latin Alexander Trallianus...*, 20–4.

18 See *ibidem* 27-8 and notes.

19 'Note, however, e.g. 2.258: "ad eos (scil. neruos) quos Graeci ankilas uocant" (beside II, 539, 32: τὰς καλουμένας ἀγκυλώσεις); 2.266: "cerota de opio confecta quae et ciliogrisa Graeci uocant" (beside II, 561, 18: ἃς οἱ παλαιοὶ καὶ χιλιοχρύσους καλεῖν ἀξιοῦσιν).' *Ibidem*, 27 n. 29.

20 *Ibidem*, 27-8.

on coughing, as well as the chapters on hiccoughing, suppurations in the lung, dysentery and paralysis are missing. Also missing from Book 2 is a considerable amount of material from the end of the section on gout. Book 3 has nothing on tertian, quotidian or quartan fevers, stopping abruptly at the end of the chapters on hectic fevers.[21]

The Latin Alexander: significant omissions from the content of the Greek *Therapeutica*[22]

Book 1:   I.567-73, 'further remedies' (for epilepsy)

Book 2:   II.169-83, 'further remedies for coughing'
           II.313-19, Περὶ λυγμοῦ ('On hiccoughing')
           II.211-27, Περὶ ἐμπυηματικῶν ('On suppurations')
           II.415-39, Περὶ δυσεντερίας ('On dysentery')
           I.575-91, Περὶ παρέσεως ('On paralysis')
           II.577.1-85.24, 'additional material on gout'

Book 3:   I.371-85, Περὶ τριταίου ('On tertian fever')
           I.385-407, Περὶ ἀμφημερινοῦ ('On quotidian fever')
           I.407-39, Περὶ τεταρταίου ('On quartan fever')

The Latin Alexander contains significant sections of text that are not found in the Greek *Therapeutica*. In Book 1 of the Latin Alexander, five chapters on diseases of the nose, face, and teeth have been added. In Book 2, extensive extracts of two lost Greek works, translated into Latin, have been added. The first of these is from what was originally a work of Philumenus, a second-century physician and contemporary of Galen,[23] on dysentery and diseases of the intestine. The second is from what was originally a work of the fourth-century Greek physician Philagrius,[24] on diseases of the spleen.

---

21 See *ibidem*, 17.

22 Adapted from Langslow, *The Latin Alexander Trallianus...*, 15-16, Table 2.1 (**ed.**, **P1**, **A** and **M**), where the references in the right-hand column are to volume (I or II) and page number in Puschmann, *Alexander von Tralles...*

23 David Langslow, *Medical Latin in the Roman Empire*. (Oxford and New York, NY: Oxford University Press, 2000), 72. For Philumenus, see Jean-Marie Jacques, "Philoumenos of Alexandria (150 – 190 CE)," in Paul T. Keyser and Georgia L. Irby-Massie (Eds.), *The encyclopedia of ancient natural scientists*. (London and New York, NY: Routledge, 2008), 661-662.

24 '[A] much-cited fourth-century Greek doctor from Epirus' (Langslow, *Medical Latin...*, 72). For Philagrius, see also John Scarborough, "Philagrios of Ēpeiros (300 – 340 CE)," in Paul T. Keyser and Georgia L. Irby-Massie (Eds.), *The encyclopedia of ancient natural scientists*. (London and New York, NY: Routledge, 2008), 643-644.

The Latin Alexander: significant additions to the content of the Greek *Therapeutica*
Book 1:   1.131-5, 'Nose, face and teeth' (Lyons 1504, 26r-28r)

Book 2:   2.79-103, 'Philumenus, on the stomach and intestines'
            2.79: *De reumate ventris Filominis*[25] [*sic*] (Lyons 1504, 47r)
            2.104-50, 'Philagrius, on the spleen'
            2.104: *Ad splenem Philagrius* (Lyons 1504, 53r)

One good indicator that Simon was utilising the Greek *Therapeutica* would be if there were any entries in the *Clavis sanationis* that could be identified as being taken only from those sections in the Greek text that are completely absent from the Latin Alexander. Evidence that Simon has used only the Latin Alexander would be if entries in the *Clavis sanationis* were to be found exclusively in those sections of the Latin Alexander that are not present in the Greek *Therapeutica*: for example in the Philumenus and Philagrius sections, and the glosses. A third possibility is that Simon has primarily used the Latin Alexander and then supplemented an entry with additional information acquired from the Greek *Therapeutica*.

I have identified many entries in the *Clavis sanationis* that are taken from the extensive extracts from Philumenus and Philagrius which have been incorporated into Book 2 of the Latin Alexander (please see Appendices 3 and 4 for details of these). One of these entries, *acantis egyptia* (where *akanthos* (ἄκανθος) is 'Bear's-foot'),[26] contains another explicit reference to the '*Practica* of Alexander' (i.e., the Latin Alexander):

Acantis egyptia (Transcript A, 1510, last accessed 12.03.12)
Acantis egyptia invenitur **in practica Alexandri** *in confectione collirii ad tingenda leucemata puto quod sit idem quod achantis arabica.*

Acantis egyptia (Print B, 1473)
Achantis egiptiaca [sic] *inuenitur* **in pratica** [sic] **Ale**. *in confectione colirii* [sic] *ad tingenda leucomata puto quod sit idem quod achantis ara.*

Egyptian *acantis* is found **in the *Practica* of Alexander** in a preparation of an eye salve for bathing white spots [white corneal opacities]. I think that it is the same as Arabic *acantis*.

---

25 In my transcriptions, where the witnesses print 'u' or 'v', I have printed 'u' or 'v' respectively throughout.
26 See Lily Y. Beck, *Pedanius Dioscorides of Anazarbus: De materia medica* (2nd edn). (Hildesheim, Zürich and New York, NY: Olms-Weidmann, 2011), 186 (Dioscorides III.17).

Furthermore, this particular entry represents an example of Simon's use of *only* the Latin Alexander. I would like to detail the method used to verify this, partly in order to illustrate the complexity in locating the exact source of Simon's information, but mainly to serve as an example of an investigation which did briefly raise the prospect that Simon *had* used the Greek *Therapeutica*.

To identify where in the Latin Alexander 'Egyptian *acantis*' is to be found, I used Opsomer's invaluable *Index de la pharmacopée du Ier au Xe siècle*[27], which lists three entries for '*Acanthus Aegyptia*' in the Lyons 1504 edition - in Book 2, Chapters 79, 80 and 98 - all of which are in the Philumenus section of the Latin Alexander; and one entry for '*Acanthi Aegyptiae Semen*', in Book 2, Chapter 123 - the Philagrius section:

Latin Alexander [Philumenus] 2.79: *De reumate ventris Filominis* [sic] (Lyons 1504, 47r-48v)
48r: *acantis*[28] *egiptiace* [sic][29]

Latin Alexander [Philumenus] 2.80: *De dissinteria reumatica* (Lyons 1504, 48v-49r)
48v: *achantem*[30] *egyptiam*[31]

Latin Alexander [Philumenus] 2.98: *Enema ad dissintericos et dolores nimios vel inflammationes* (Lyons 1504, 51v-52r)
52r: *achanthos*[32] *egyptie*[33]

Latin Alexander [Philagrius] 2.123: *De fomentationibus* (Lyons 1504, 55r-55v)
55v: *egyptie*[34] *acautis* [sic][35] *semen*

---

27 Carmelia Opsomer, *Index de la pharmacopée du Ier au Xe siècle*, 2 vols. (Hildesheim, Zürich and New York, NY: Olms-Weidmann, 1989).

28 + gloss 'l': '*id est spine albe.*' (48r).

29 Cf. Peter Mihăileanu, *Fragmentele latine ale lui Philumenus și Philagrius*. (Bucharest: Institutul de Arte Grafice 'Carol Göbl', 1910), 110.7: *acantis aegyptias* [+ variants]; cf. Theodor Puschmann, *Nachträge zu Alexander Trallianus: Fragmente aus Philumenus und Philagrius* (repr. 1963, Amsterdam: A. M. Hakkert), (Berlin: S. Calvary and Co., 1886), 24: *acanthi Aegyptiacae* [no variants].

30 + gloss 'c': '*id est spinam al(_)s.*' (48v).

31 Cf. Mihăileanu, *Fragmentele latine...*, 116.10: *acantem egyptiam* [+ variants]; cf. Puschmann, *Nachträge zu Alexander Trallianus...*, 32: *acanthum Aegyptiacam* [no variants].

32 + gloss 'z': '*id est spine albe.*' (52r).

33 Cf. Mihăileanu, *Fragmentele latine...*, 139.11: *acantis egyptias* [+ variants]; cf. Puschmann, *Nachträge zu Alexander Trallianus...*, 62: *acanthi Aegyptiae* [no variants].

34 + gloss 'm': '*id est spine albe.*' (55v).

35 Cf. Mihăileanu, *Fragmentele latine...*, 165.2: *aegyptiae acantis* [+ variants]; cf. Puschmann, *Nachträge zu Alexander Trallianus...*, 96: *Aegyptiae acanthi* [no variants].

The entry in Simon for 'Egyptian *acantis*', however, refers to 'an eye salve for bathing white spots' – '*leucomata*'. Therefore none of these four entries, found in the Philumenus and Philagrius sections of the Latin Alexander - on dysentery and diseases of the intestine, and diseases of the spleen respectively - are Simon's source. Perhaps this example could have been taken from the Greek *Therapeutica*. A TLG[36] lemma search of the Greek *Therapeutica* for 'λευκωμα' yields three results,[37] one of which is a recipe for 'white spots/*leucomata*' (Πρὸς τὸ βάψαι λευκώματα λίαν καλόν; 'For 'dyeing' white spots, a very good [treatment]', II.51.1), which does indeed contain ἀκάνθης Αἰγυπτίας (II.51.3). Furthermore, this particular recipe is *not* found in the Latin Alexander. Has Simon used the Greek *Therapeutica* for this entry? Further investigation indicates not. Closer examination of the section in the Lyons 1504 edition of the Latin Alexander that is equivalent to this section of the Greek *Therapeutica* – within the chapters dealing with eye salves ('*colliria*') - reveals an entry in the Latin Alexander that does correspond to Simon's entry: Book 1, Chapter 101 '*Ad tingendas albugines et leucomata tingenda*' (Lyons 1504, 21r), and a recipe which contains '*anchotis*[38] egyptie [sic]'.[39] This particular chapter heading and recipe are not found in the Greek *Therapeutica* (II.49). Indeed, to date, I have been unable to identify any entries in the *Clavis sanationis* that are to be found only in Alexander's Greek *Therapeutica* and not in the Latin Alexander.

One thing that is noticeable from the study of 'Egyptian *acantis*' is the variation/error in spelling. Indeed, spelling variations/errors abound both between traditions and within traditions. I would like to use Simon's entry for *orodes humores* - an entry which refers to glosses found in the Latin Alexander - to illustrate the difference between Print A and Print B of the *Clavis sanationis*:

Orodes humores (Transcript A, 1510, last accessed 13.02.12)
Orodes humores .i. serosi aquosi ut Alex. ca. de nausea. Item ca. de scabie vesice. Item ca. de catarticis podagricorum, evocant inquit tenues humores quos greci orodes vocant, interdum oroides invenitur ab oros quod est serum lactis.

Orodes humores (Print B, 1473)
Orodes humores .i. serosi aquosi ut Alex ca. de nausea item ca. de catarticis podagriorum [sic] euacuant inquit tenues humores quos gr(_). or(o)des uocant interdum oriodes [sic] inuenitur ab oros quod est serum lactis.

---

36 *Thesaurus Linguae Graecae*: http://www.tlg.uci.edu/
37 2 × λευκώματα, II.37.7 and II.51.1; 1 × λευκωμάτων, II.31.15.
38 + gloss 'a': '*id est spine nigre*.' [sic] (21r).
39 '*Giptias*' in Angers, *Bibl. mun.* 457 (34ra), using Langslow's transcript.

Orodes humores, that is serous, aqueous, as in the chapter of Alexander 'On nausea'; likewise in his chapter 'On cathartics for gout'. They evacuate, he says, thin humours, which the Greeks call *orodes*. Occasionally the spelling *oriodes* [*sic*] is found. [The word originates] from *oros*, which is the whey of milk. (Translating Print B, 1473)

As is noted by Langslow[40], Greek ὀρ[ρ]ώδης (Latin *orodes*) is given a 'rudimentary' etymology in the Latin Alexander at 2.42 – this is Simon's chapter 'Cn nausea' (*ca. de nausea*), and occurs twice more at 2.249[41] – this is Simon's chapter 'On cathartics for gout' (*ca. de catarticis podagri[c]orum*).

Note that Print A of the *Clavis sanationis* also includes the reference 'likewise in the chapter 'On itchiness of the bladder'' (*Item ca. de scabie vesice*), which is also found in Print C (1486). Print B, however, and Manuscript **e** (*Laur. plut.* 73, cod. 31) both omit mention of this particular chapter. This is quite possibly a case of *saut du même au même* – the eye leaping from *item* to *item* – however, I suspect the reason might be more complex.

The additional chapter reference found in Print A and Print C is to Book 2, Chapter 198 of the Latin Alexander, which is in a section that is also found in the Greek (II.491.11 ff.). As with the 'Egyptian *acantis*' example above, there was a brief glimmer that perhaps Simon did have access to and was using a Greek text after all. However, consider the following:

Latin Alexander 2.198: *Curatio eiusdem*[42]
Est autem confectio medicaminis quod facit **ad orodes**[i] [ms. **A** = *ad sorodis*, for Greek ψωρώδεις[43]] *passiones et dissurias inflammationes renum et vesice sanat / sed et ulcera vesice cum flegmone f(a)cta(m) sanat.* (Lyons 1504, 68v)

There is moreover a preparation of a medicament which is effective against *orodes* diseases and it cures painful urination [and] inflammations of the kidneys and bladder, but also it cures ulcers of the bladder with inflammation.

---

40 Langslow, *The Latin Alexander Trallianus...*, 28 and n. 31

41 'At 2.249, first it is glossed with Latin *aquosus*, then in the very next sentence it recurs in a *quod Graeci uocant* formula, where Puschmann's text has not ὀρρώδης but λεπτός: 2.249: "*dandum est catarticum quod possit educere pingue et spissum flegma et non orode id est aquosum et tenue urinae simile, quemadmodum multi faciunt dantes lacterides et opos tit mali et cnidium coccum admiscentes et sic euacuant tenuiores humores quos Graeci orodes uocant*" (II, 521, 5-7: τὸ δυνάμενον ἑλκῦσαι παχὺ φλέγμα καὶ ὀρρῶδες, ὥσπερ ποιοῦσι πολλοὶ λαθυρίδας τε καὶ ὀπὸν τιθυμάλλου καὶ Κνίδιον κόκκον παρέχοντες αὐτοῖς, οἳ τὰ λεττὰ κενοῦντες ῥεύματα).' Langslow, *The Latin Alexander Trallianus...*, 28 and n. 31.

42 Where 2.197 is *Si vesica scabiosa sit*; the same chapter title is found in **G2** and **L1**; **P1** and [ms.] **A** have *Signa si uesica scabra sit, Ibidem*, 251.

43 Puschmann, *Alexander von Tralles...*, II.493.4

As can be seen, Lyons 1504 (68v) has '***ad orodes***[i]' which even includes the gloss '**i**': *id est serosas seu aquosas* (68v). However, the eleventh-century manuscript Angers, *Bibl. mun.* 457, Langslow's **A**, has *sorodis*, a transliteration of Greek ψωρώδεις.[44] Possibly, Simon had a corrupt exemplar with the reading *orodes*, which is transmitted in Print A and Print C - hence the extra reference – and then, possibly, someone has spotted the error with the result that Print B and Manuscript **e** represent a corrected version.

As another example of spelling errors, consider Simon's entry for *embalmata* (that is, *emba**m**mata*, 'sauces'):[45]

> *Embalmata* (Transcript A, 1510, last accessed 12.03.12, entry edited by Barbara Zipser)
> *Embalmata Alexan. ca. de medicinis ad frigidum stomachum, item de reumatismo ventris sunt intinctiones seu salsamenta in quibus morselli intinguntur.*
> *Embasmata* AC | *Embalmata* B e | *iunctiones* A | *intinctiones* B e | *inunctiones* C

According to Alexander, [in the] chapter on medicines for a cold stomach, also [in the chapter] on flux from the belly, *embalmata* are dips or sauces in which bits of food are dipped.

The second chapter referred to in this entry, 'On flux from the belly' ('*de reumatismo ventris*'), is to be found in Book 2 of the Latin Alexander, Chapter 79[46] - the 'Philumenus' section:

> Latin Alexander 2.79: *De reumate ventris Filominis* [sic] (Lyons 1504, 47r-48v)
> 48r: *Item embalmata*[47][48] [ms. **A** = *bamata*] *hoc modo ad hoc conficiuntur. Cimino cum salis modico et aceto oleo confecto intingitur quod edendum est.*

---

44 LSJ: 'of the nature of the itch, scabby'. '[I]n Cassius Felix ... *scabiosus* is synonymous with Greek *psoricus*, it means "for treating *scabies*" ...', Langslow, *Medical Latin in the Roman Empire*, 344.

45 OLD: *embamma, atis* (n.) [Gk. ἔμβαμμα] = '[a] sauce or dressing for food, esp. one made with vinegar'.

46 Cf. Puschmann, *Nachträge zu Alexander Trallianus...*, 26: *Item embammata hoc modo ad hoc conficiuntur. Cymino cum sale et modico aceto et oleo confecto intingitur quod edendum est. ... Potest autem iuvare et scorpio piscis assatus et cum cymini praedicti embammate datus et ostreae in suis* [+ n. 61, re. variant *sibi*] *testis assatae et sumptae.* Cf. also Mihăileanu, *Fragmentele latine...*, 112, 8-16: *Item embammata hoc modo ad haec conficiuntur: cimino cum salis modico et aceto et oleo confecto intingitur, quod edendum est. ... Potest enim iuvare et scorpion piscis assus* [+ variants: *assa* and *assatus*] *et cum cimini praedicti embammate datus et ostreae in suis testis assatae et assumptae* [+ variants: *adsumta, sumpta* and *sumptae*].

47 + gloss 'c': '*sunt intinctiones seu salse* [sic] *in quibus morselli intinguntur. ian(_).*' (48r).

48 Cf. Mihăileanu, *Fragmentele latine...*, 112.8: *embammata* [no variants]; cf. Puschmann, *Nachträge zu Alexander Trallianus...*, 26: *embammata* [no variants].

48v: *Potest autem iuuare et scorpio piscis assatus et cum cimini praedicti embalmate*[49][50] *datus et ostree in suis testis assate et sumpte.*

48r: Likewise *embalmata* are prepared in the following way. What is to be eaten is dipped in cumin prepared in oil with a modicum of salt and uinegar.

48v: Moreover scorpion fish, roasted and given with an *embalma* of the aforementioned cumin is also able to help, and oysters roasted in their own shells and eaten.

The first chapter, however, 'On medicines for a cold stomach' ('*de medicinis ad frigidum stomachum*'), is to be found in Book 2, Chapter 46, of the Latin Alexander – *not* a 'Philumenus' section:

Latin Alexander 2.46: *Ad frigidum stomachum embalmata*[51] (Lyons 1504, 40v) [ms. **A** = *inbamata*]
40v: [*E*]*mbalmata* ... [for Greek ἔμβαμμα [*sic*]][52]

Moreover, it is also found in Book II of the Greek *Therapeutica*. It is important to note, however, that whereas in the Latin we have *embalmata*, in the Greek we have ἔμβαμμα.[53]

The following is taken from the entry for *embalmata* in *Simon Online*:

... The apparatus of Puschmann's edition does not list any variant readings in this heading. ... Most likely, the error was caused by a Greek manuscript: in Greek minuscule, the letters μ and λ ('m' and 'l') look very similar and can easily be confused; in majuscule, M looks like a double Λ. An unknown scribe or translator mistook a 'm' for an 'l', erroneously assuming the word was in fact derived from ἐμβάλλειν /emballein/ 'to put inside'.[54]

---

49 + gloss 'a': '*id est salsamente.*' (48v).
50 Cf. Mihăileanu, *Fragmentele latine...*, 112.15: *embammate* [no variants]; cf. Puschmann, *Nachträge zu Alexander Trallianus...*, 26: *embammate* [no variants].
51 + gloss 'f': '*sunt intinctiones seu salsamenta in quibus morselli intinguntur. Ian(_).*' (40v).
52 Πρὸς κατεψυγμένον στόμαχον ἔμβαμμα - Puschmann, *Alexander von Tralles...*, II.305.27.
53 Πρὸς κατεψυγμένον στόμαχον ἔμβαμμα. | Ἀρκευθίδων οὐγγ. β´ | πεπέρεως οὐγγ. β´ | ζιγγιβέρεως οὐγγ. δ´ | πετροσελίνου οὐγ. α´ | μέλιτος τὸ ἀρκοῦν. | χρῶ ὡς καλλίστῳ. Ibidem, II.305.27-33.
54 *embalmata*: *Simon Online*, last accessed 12.03.12, entry edited by Barbara Zipser

As can be seen in the three entries from the *Clavis sanationis* discussed in detail above - *acantis egyptia*, *embalmata* (that is, *emba**m**mata*) and *orodes humores* – spelling errors/variants can be very misleading. They can also be very useful. Indeed, a close study of these errors/variants, as well as additions and omissions, found when comparing Simon's *Clavis sanationis* with the Latin Alexander might make it possible to narrow down Simon's manuscript source or sources, and potentially assign them to a particular branch of Langslow's stemma (given in Appendix 2, and reproduced with the kind permission of David Langslow). For example, the fact that Simon often quotes from those sections of the Latin Alexander that we know are in fact interpolations from the translated works of Philumenus and Philagrius (Appendices 3 and 4), without referring to Philagrius or Philumenus by name, is potentially useful.

In the Lyons 1504 edition of the Latin Alexander, Chapter 2.79, 'On flux from the belly', is clearly headed 'On flux from the belly, of Philumenus' (*De reumate ventris Filominis* [*sic*], 47r), as indeed it is in the manuscripts **G2, L1, P1** (*De reuma* ...) and **A**.[55] Furthermore, a later chapter, Chapter 2.81, 'Signs of dysentery', is also identified as by Philumenus (*Signa dissinterice passionis Philomini*) in Lyons 1504 (49r), and in the manuscripts **G2, L1** and **A**, and although Philumenus is not mentioned in the title here in **P1**, the chapter begins with 'Of Philumenus' (*Filomini*).[56] The same is seen in the heading for Chapter 2.99, 'On bowel diseases, of Philumenus' (*De ciliacis* [i.e., *coeliacis*] *Philomini*), with the title in Lyons 1504 (52r) and the manuscripts **G2, L1** and **A** all mentioning Philumenus, but with the chapter in **P1** beginning, this time with an error, '*Flaminum*' [*sic*].[57]

Likewise in Lyons 1504, Chapter 2.104 is clearly headed 'Philagrius on the spleen' (*Ad splenem Philagrius*, 53r), as indeed it is in the manuscripts **G2, L1** and **A**; here **P1** has no title.[58] Furthermore, the chapter heading of 2.151 on dropsy, immediately following the end of the Philagrius section, (*Causa que est ydropicie Alexandri*, Lyons 1504, 59r), is explicitly assigned to Alexander, clearly signalling the return to his work. This explicit reference to Alexander is also seen in the equivalent chapter headings in **G2, L1, P1** and **A**.[59]

Given that Simon's entries contain no reference to Philumenus or Philagrius, one does have to wonder whether Simon's exemplar(s) contained the overt references to Philumenus and Philagrius.

---

55 Langslow, *The Latin Alexander Trallianus...*, 246.
56 *Ibidem*, 246.
57 *Ibidem*.
58 *Ibidem*.
59 **P1**: '*Causa aedropiciae alexandriae*'; [ms.] **A**: '*Causa ydropicie Alexandri*' - *Ibidem*, 249.

Consider again the excerpt taken from the moderately lengthy entry for *sauich* and the reference to the fact that in books translated from the Greek, '*sauich*' is written '*polenta*':

Sauich (Print B, 1473)
... notandum tamen quod ubicumque habetur in liberis [sic] de arabico translatis sauich apud Dia. et Alex. et Paul(_) et alios de greco translatos habetur **polenta** *quare secudum [sic] idem uidetur apud grecos uero uocatur alfita ut patet per Gal(_). ca. de alfitis in libro de alimentis item Ste. in sinonimis dicit quod alfiton est sauich.*

... Note, however, that everywhere it is written in books translated from Arabic [it is] *sauich*; in the writings of Dioscorides and Alexander and Paul and others translated from the Greek, it is written **polenta**, for which reason we may assume they are synonyms. Among the Greeks, indeed, it is called *alphita*, as is revealed through Galen in the chapter on *alphita* in his book *On foods*. Likewise Stephanus in his *Synonyms* says that *alphita* is *sauich*.

Opsomer[60] records just one occurrence of *polenta* in the Latin Alexander, in Book 3, Chapter 66, *Lixoperita epithimata et embroce et emplastra febrientibus Martyrii medici*[61] (Lyons 1504, 92v-93r):

93r: *Item embroca ex alica*[62] *aut oxilapatos*[63] *autem bene facit et succus si de polenta .i. alfita*[64] *tenui modicum ei misces infuso duplicato panno molli.*

If Simon's reference to 'Alexander' and '*polenta*' does in fact refer to Book 3, Chapter 66, it is referring to a section in the Latin Alexander that is not found in many of the Latin manuscripts,[65] and has no equivalent in Puschmann's Greek text.[66] [67] [68] Moreover, even where this chapter *is* found in the Latin manuscripts, it is not always present in its entirety.

---

60 Carmelia Opsomer, *Index de la pharmacopée...*
61 See Langslow, *The Latin Alexander Trallianus...*, 262 n. 110 for variants.
62 + gloss 'e': '*alica est genus frumenti quidam speltam putant.*' (93r).
63 + gloss 'f': '*id est acetosa herba.*' (93r).
64 + gloss 'g': '*id est farina ordei.*' (93r).
65 Langslow, *The Latin Alexander Trallianus...*, 59.
66 Puschmann, *Alexander von Tralles...*
67 '... 3.66 ... is not in the Greek Alexander as we have it, and ... could be an addition to the original version of the *Latin Alexander...*' – Langslow, *The Latin Alexander Trallianus...*, 58.
68 However, compare the Latin found at Lyons 1504, 93r (*Item embroca ex alica aut oxilapatos autem bene facit et succus si de polenta .i. alfita tenui modicum ei misces infuso*

The whole chapter is missing from **P1, A, O, D, Ox, Ge, Ma, P2, L2** and **B**.[69] It is present in **M, G1, Mu, C, P3, G2, L1** and, of course, Lyons 1504 (Langslow's ***ed.***).[70] Of itself, this is not proof that Simon used this manuscript or that manuscript, not least because I am not absolutely sure that this chapter is the source of Simon's comment on *polenta*.

Consider now three entries in the *Clavis sanationis* – *amitrocera*, *centron* and *acros* - all of which occur in the chapters on coughing at the beginning of Book 2 of the Latin Alexander; chapters, moreover, which are to be found in Langslow's published edition with a full apparatus.[71]

---

duplicato panno molli) with the following three extracts of Greek texts taken from Galen, Oribasius and Aëtius: [1.] Galen (*De methodo medendi* 10.9, C. G. Kühn, *Claudii Galeni opera omnia*, vol. 10 (repr. 1965, Hildesheim: Olms, Leipzig: Knobloch, 1825)): Ἄλλο φάρμακον. **ὀξαλίδος ἢ ὀξυλαπάθου χυλὸς**, ἀλφίτων λεπτῶν ὀλίγων μιχθέντων ἀναλαμβανέσθω διπτύχῳ ῥάκει τριβακῷ, ψυχρὸν δ' ἱκανῶς ἐπιτιθέσθω καὶ τοῦτο. μὴ παρόντος δὲ τοιούτου ῥάκους, ὀθόνιον δίπτυχον ἀναδεύσας, ἐπιτίθει τῷ ψύχεσθαι δεομένῳ μορίῳ); [2.] Oribasius (*Collectiones medicae* 44.24.17): **Ὀξαλίδος ἢ ὀξυλαπάθου χυλὸς** ἀλφίτων ὀλίγων μιχθέντων ἀναλαμβανέσθω διπτύχῳ ῥάκει ἢ ὀθονίῳ· ψυχρὸν δ' ἱκανῶς ἐπιτιθέσθω; [3.] Aëtius: (*Iatricorum liber* 5.92.97-9): ἄλλο ἐπίθεμα κάλλιστον. **ὀξυλαπάθου χυλῷ** ἀλφίτων λεπτῶν μιχθέντων ἀναλαμβανέσθω διπτύχῳ ῥάκει τριβακῷ καὶ ψυχρὸν ἐπιτιθέσθω. Note especially that, whereas both Galen and Oribasius have ὀξαλίδος ἢ ὀξυλαπάθου [χυλὸς], Aëtius has only ὀξυλαπάθου [χυλῷ]. There are further textual resonances between the Latin text of chapter 3.66 and the Greek texts of Galen, Oribasius and Aëtius. Indeed, elsewhere in chapter 3.66 we find overt references to both Galen ('*Emplastrum Galieni* ...', 92v) and Oribasius ('*Item lixoperitum Oribasii* ...', 93r). Furthermore, the '*lixoperitum Oribasii*' found in 3.66 of the Latin Alexander is strikingly similar to the '*lyxypyreton* [sic] ... *mirabilem*' of the Latin Oribasius at *Synopsis* 3.60 (see Ulco Cats Bussemaker, Charles Daremberg and Auguste Molinier, *Oeuvres d'Oribase*, 6 vols. (Paris: Imprimerie Nationale, 1851-76), 5.863), which itself is to be found in the Greek Oribasius (Johann Raeder, *Oribasii synopsis ad Eustathium et libri ad Eunapium* [*Corpus medicorum Graecorum* 6.3] (repr. 1964, Amsterdam: A. M. Hakkert, Leipzig: Teubner, 1926), 3.60.

69 See Langslow, *The Latin Alexander Trallianus*..., 40 (for **A**: 'text breaking off abruptly in 3.34'); 41 (for **B**: 'just less than half a page of the start of Book 3'); 42 (for **D**: 'text of Book 3, to end of 3.65'); 43 (for **Ge**: 'text of 3.1-65'); 45 (for **L2**: 'unnumbered chapters ending with the end of 3.65' and **Ma**: 'text of 3.1-65'); 48 (for **O**: 'text, breaking off abruptly after (3.13 *ad fin.*) ...'); 49 (for **Ox**: 'expl. 119r (end of 3.65) ...'); 50 (for **P1**: 'text of Book 3, breaking off at 3.63 ...' and **P2**: 'text of Book 3, ending with 3.65').

70 See Langslow, *The Latin Alexander Trallianus*..., 42 (for **C**: 'text of Book 3, including all but the very last recipe of 3.66'); 44 (for **G1**: 'text of Book 3, including all but the very last recipe of 3.66', **G2**: 'Book 3 ... 66 chapters' and **L1**: 'Book 3 ... 66 ... chapters'); 46 (for **M**: 'Book 3 ending with the penultimate recipe of 3.66 (minus the last three words)') and 47 (for **Mu**: 'text of Book 3 to the very end of 3.66'); 51 (for **P3**: 'text of Book 3, breaking off without an Explicit after only 8 lines of 3.66 ...').

71 Langslow, The Latin Alexander Trallianus..., 175-229.

First, *amitrocera*, which has the following entry in Simon:

Amitrocera (Transcript A, 1510, last accessed 10.03.12)

Amitrocera .g. facilis ad cognoscendum. Alexan. ca. de tussi materialis autem et cetera.

Amitrocera (Print B, 1473)

Amicrotera [sic] gr(_). facilis ad cognoscendum Alex. capitulo de tussi materialis et cetera.

The following text, relevant apparatus and translation of the Latin Alexander is taken from Langslow:[72][73]

2.4.2 Differunt igitur quod magis operatiu*ae* habent manifestas significationes, material*es* autem [si accesserit tussis] amitroter*as* {for Greek **ἀμυδρότερα**[74]},[75] et non oportet <t>alia[76] iterum dicere.

amitroter*as scripsimus* (*fort. cf.* a materi*a est* **M**)] -a ***plerique*** (amet- **P1** amyt- **P2** amicr- **G2 L1**) amitro terea **O** amicio tera ***ed.***[77] amitrota **Ge** a materia **M** *om.* **Mu** (*post* a. *habent* est **M D P3** *add.* **m3**) **G2**

---

72 See Langslow, *The Latin Alexander Trallianus...*, 200-3. Where {...} indicates additional material.

73 Cf. Lyons 1504, 32v: *Differunt igitur quod operatiue* [+ gloss 'g': *id est actine qualitates*] *magis manifestas habent significationes. Cap( ). 5: De tussi si ex humoribus fiat. [M]aterialis autem si accesserit tussis amicio* [+ gloss 'h': *id est facilis ad cognoscendum. Ian(_).*] *tera* [+ gloss 'i': *est* [sic]] *et non oportet iterum taliter dici* [+ gloss 'k': *.s. signa quibus cognoscatur si materialis est*]. Langslow notes that, in an 'apparent corruption common to all the Latin manuscripts', '*si accesserit tussis*' has been added 'in an effort to make sense of a Latin text rendered unintelligible by the transposition of the section-heading 2.5.t. *De tusse si ex humoribus fiat* (itself not in the Greek text either)', Langslow, *The Latin Alexander Trallianus...*, 104.

74 Puschmann, *Alexander von Tralles...*, II.149.13

75 Langslow, *The Latin Alexander Trallianus...*, 117: 'The Latin tradition offers various explanatory notes to Greek ἀμυδρότερα, among which P2 and B alone have *leuior ad curandum*, and G1 alone the very similar *leuis ad curandum*. [+ n. 18: 'cf. *leuior facilior ad curandum* Ma *.i. leuis* P3 m3(?) *.i. facilis ad cognoscendum* Ox Φ']. Langslow, *The Latin Alexander Trallianus...*, 129: 'Ox and Φ also transpose *efficitur* and *tussis*.'

76 Where the reading '<t>alia' is to be credited to Cloudy Fischer.

77 Where Langslow's ***ed.*** = Lyons 1504.

They differ in that the active tend rather to have clear signs, while the material ones have more indistinct signs. And it is not necessary to say this again.

The following is Langslow's note on *amitroteras*:[78]

amitroteras ... ἀμυδρός 'faint' is transliterated also at 1.59 '*Pulsus etiam raros et breues et amidros habent*' (= I, 529, 11 καὶ τοὺς σφυγμοὺς ἀραιοὺς καὶ μικροὺς καὶ ἀμυδροὺς ἴσχουσιν) and 3.41 (I, 345, 25); cf. 3.45 (I, 347, 21) where ἀμυδρός is confused with ἄμετρος and translated *absque mensura*. That the word was less than familiar is seen clearly at 3.48 '*pulsus ... paruus autem et amidros in ethica febre*', where the Latin version adds the note: '*Amidros autem pulsus dicitur defectus, qui solutam habet uirtutem et percussionem facit imbecillem*'. (The marginal gloss at this point ... reads '*.i. imbecillis seu debilis. Gal. in lib. de differentiis febrium*'.)[79]

Of interest here are those manuscripts that *do not* include *amitrocera* – regardless of spelling - that is: **M, Mu** and **Ge**.

Secondly *centron*, which has the following entry in Simon:

Centron (Transcript A, 1510, last accessed 10.03.12)

Centron Alex. ca. tussi exponunt quidam punctiones.

Centron (Print B, 1473)

Ceneron [sic] *Alexan. ca. de tussi exponit quedam* [sic] *punctiones.*

Again, the following text, relevant apparatus and translation is taken from Langslow:[80]

2.9.2 Et spuunt nihil, neque soni aliquid aut cencron {for Greek κέρχνον[81]} patiuntur. Neque enim contingere poterit [nisi] ex indigesto et necdum permixto *fymate*.

---

78 Langslow, *The Latin Alexander Trallianus...*, 201 n.85.

79 Cf. Simon (Transcript A, 1510, last accessed 12.03.12) '*Amidros: Amidros pulsus Alex. capitulo de litargia exponitur a .G. liber de doctrina pulsuum quod est imbecillis seu debilis. Sed liber de doctrina greca amidron obscurum minus apparens.*'

80 Langslow, *The Latin Alexander Trallianus...*, 216-17. Cf. Lyons 1504, 33r: *Et spuunt nihil: neque soni aliquid aut centron* [sic + gloss 'h': *centron exponunt quidam punctiones*] *patiuntur. Neque enim contingere* [+ gloss 'i': *tussis .s. vel centron*] *potest nisi ex indigestione et nedum* [sic] *permixto fimate* [+ gloss 'k': *id est inflato(_)e turge(_)te vel pusculosa vel tuberculo. Ian(_).*].

81 Puschmann, *Alexander von Tralles...*, II.153.2

cencron **P3**] concron **Ma** centron *cett*. cetron **Mu** cendron **O** centro **A** centrum **P1** tenorum **M** *ad hoc uerbum habent* .i. punccionem **Ma** .i. punctionem **D** centron exponunt quidam punctiones Φ

And they spit nothing up, nor do they suffer any noise (in the ears) or hoarseness, for it cannot possibly occur while the tumour is immature and not yet thoroughly mixed.

Langslow's note on *cencron* is as follows:

cencron The Latin variants suggest Greek κέγχρος, which means 'millet', rather than κέρχνος 'roughness, hoarseness', which is very suitably rendered with *raucor* in the very next section (2.10.1). LSJ, s. vv., suggests some confusion between the two Greek words, attesting κέρχνος 'millet' but not κέγχρος 'hoarseness'.[82]

What is important in this example are the glosses added to **Ma**, **D** and Φ, given that Simon Print A has '*exponunt quidam punctiones*' and Simon Print B has '*exponit quedam* [sic] *punctiones*', where *punctiones* are 'stabbing pains'. Thirdly, Simon's entry for *acros*:

Acros (Transcript A, 1510, last accessed 15.03.12)

Acros .i. acredo Alex. capitulo de tussi, quando aut de subito et cetera.

Acros (Print B, 1473)

Acros .i. acredo Alex. capitulo de tussi quando autem subito et cetera.

Once again, the following text and relevant apparatus is taken from Langslow:[83]

2.10.1 Quando autem desubito qui laborant sentiunt coangustata praecordia se habere et absque febribus molestari et sit*i* mult*a*, *sed* habent etiam quendam raucorem {for Greek κέρχνον[84] } cum tusse ...

---

82 Langslow, *The Latin Alexander Trallianus...*, 216 n. 157.
83 Langslow, *The Latin Alexander Trallianus...*, 218-19. Cf. Lyons 1504, 33r: *[A]liquando autem de subito qui laborant sentiunt p(rae)angustata* [sic] *p(rae)cordia se habere et absque febribus molestari: et sitis multa sit / et habent etiam quandam* [sic] *rancorem* [sic] *et acrorem cum tusse ...*
84 Puschmann, *Alexander von Tralles...*, II.153.9.

raucorem **O L2 P3** (ruccorem **P1** rugura **M**)] ranc(h)orem ***cett***. |*ante* cum *habent* et acrorem **P3 D Ox Ge G2 *ed.*** acrorem **Ma**

When the patients suddenly feel that the chest is constricted and troubled (although) without fever and without great thirst, but they have also a certain hoarseness with the cough ...

Here, it is the addition of *et acrorem* before *raucorem*, seen in the manuscripts **P3, D, Ox, Ge, G2** and Lyons 1504 (Langslow's **ed.**), and *acrorem* before *raucorem* in the manuscript **Ma** which is interesting. *acror* is 'a bitter taste in the mouth', hence Simon's *id est acredo*, where *acredo* is 'a sharp or pungent taste'. There is no equivalent to this in Puschmann's Greek text.[85]

By collecting further examples, more evidence could be found that perhaps might indeed help locate Simon's source or sources on Langslow's stemma. So far, based on the evidence of *amitrocera, centron* and *acros*, Φ has 'three ticks', but the tradition above is very complex and therefore care must be taken before positing any firm conclusions. However, the shared innovations between both Simon and Φ are striking.[86]

In this paper, I hope to have showed that Simon, when compiling his *Clavis sanationis*, used the Latin Alexander. I have also made a tentative first attempt to locate Simon's exemplar(s) on David Langslow's stemma. I would like to end with a brief comment on the Lyons 1504 edition of the Latin Alexander, the *Practica Alexandri yatros greci cum expositione glose interlinearis Iacobi de partibus et Ianuensis in margine posite* – to give it its full title - edited by Fr. Fradin. The '*Iacobus de partibus*' of the title is Jacques Despars (*c.* 1380-1458)[87] and the '*Ianuensis*' is '[*Simonis*] *Ianuensis*' - Simon of Genoa. The Lyons 1504 edition includes a vast number of glosses that represent the scholarly endeavours of both Jacques Despars and Simon of Genoa (throughout this paper, whenever I have quoted from the Lyons 1504 edition of the Latin Alexander, I have included a reference to any glosses in the footnotes). In conclusion, therefore, not only is the Latin Alexander a 'source text' for Simon's *Clavis sanationis*, but also the entries in the *Clavis sanationis* that are taken from the Latin Alexander are of great importance for any consideration of the Lyons 1504 printed edition, as well as the extremely complex later manuscript tradition of the Latin Alexander.

---

85 Puschmann, *Alexander von Tralles*....

86 For the 'Φ-recension' and 'sources of Φ', see Langslow, *The Latin Alexander Trallianus...*, 126-30.

87 For Jacques Despars, see Thomas Glick, Steven Livesey, and Wallis (Eds.), *Medieval science, technology and medicine: An encyclopedia.* (New York, NY: Routledge, 2005), 151-2; Langslow, *The Latin Alexander Trallianus...*,10 and n. 77.

Bibliography

Primary sources, early printed books and manuscripts:

Alexander Trallianus: *Practica Alexandri yatros greci cum expositione glose interlinearis Iacobi de partibus et Ianuensis in margine posite*, edited by Fr. Fradin. Lyons 1504.

S mon Print A = *Simonis Januensis opusculum cui nomen Clavis sanationis simplicia medicinalia latina greca at arabica ordine alphabetico mirifice elucidans recognitum ac mendis purgatum et quotationibus Plinii maxime: ac aliorum in marginibus ornatum.* Venice: For heirs of O. Scotus by B. Locatellus, 1510.

S mon Print B = *Synonyma Simonis Genuensis, opus impressum per Antonium Zarotum parmensem.* Milano 1473.

S mon Print C = *Simon Ianuensis Clavis sanationis*, Venetiis per Gulielmum de Tridino ex Monteserato, 1486.

S mon Manuscript e = Biblioteca Medicea Laurenziana Plut. 73, cod. 31, f. 6 -110r ff.

Primary sources, other:

Bussemaker, Ulco Cats, Charles Daremberg and Auguste Molinier. *Oeuvres d Oribase*, 6 vols. Paris: Imprimerie Nationale, 1851-1876.

Heiberg, Johan Ludvig. *Pauli Aeginetae libri tertii interpretatio latina antiqua.* Leipzig: Teubner, 1912.

Kühn, C. G. *Claudii Galeni opera omnia*, vol. 10, repr. 1965, Hildesheim: Olms. Leipzig: Knobloch, 1825.

Langslow, David R. "Chapter 5: An edition of the Latin Alexander on coughing." In *idem, The Latin Alexander Trallianus: The text and transmission of a Late Latin medical book*. 175-229. London: Society for the Promotion of Roman Studies, 2006.

Masullo, Rita. *Filagrio: Frammenti*. Naples: Bibliopolis, 1999.

Mihăileanu, Peter. *Fragmentele latine ale lui Philumenus și Philagrius*. Bucharest: Institutul de Arte Grafice 'Carol Göbl', 1910.

Olivieri, Alessandro. *Aëtii Amideni libri medicinales v-viii* [*Corpus medicorum Graecorum* 8.2]. Berlin: Akademie-Verlag, 1950.

Puschmann, Theodor. *Alexander von Tralles. Original-Text und Übersetzung nebst einer einleitenden Abhandlung. Ein Beitrag zur Geschichte der Medicin*, 2 vols, repr. 1963, Amsterdam: A. M. Hakkert. Vienna: W. Braumüller, 1878-1879.

— *Nachträge zu Alexander Trallianus: Fragmente aus Philumenus und Philagrius*, repr. 1963, Amsterdam: A. M. Hakkert. Berlin: S. Calvary and Co., 1886.

Raeder, Johann. *Oribasii synopsis ad Eustathium et libri ad Eunapium* [*Corpus medicorum Graecorum* 6.3]. repr. 1964, Amsterdam: A. M. Hakkert. Leipzig: Teubner, 1926.

— *Oribasii collectionum medicarum reliquiae*, vols 1-4 [*Corpus medicorum Graecorum* 6.1.1-6.2.2]. Leipzig: Teubner, 1928-1933.

Secondary sources:

Beck, Lily Y. *Pedanius Dioscorides of Anazarbus:* De materia medica (2nd edn). Hildesheim, Zürich and New York, NY: Olms-Weidmann, 2011.

Glick, Thomas F., Steven John Livesey and Faith Wallis (Eds.). *Medieval science, technology and medicine: An encyclopedia*. New York, NY: Routledge, 2005.

Jacques, Jean-Marie. "Philoumenos of Alexandria (150 – 190 CE)." In Paul T. Keyser and Georgia L. Irby-Massie (Eds.), *The encyclopedia of ancient natural scientists*. 661-662. London and New York, NY: Routledge, 2008.

Langslow, David R. *Medical Latin in the Roman Empire*. Oxford and New York, NY: Oxford University Press, 2000.

— *The Latin Alexander Trallianus: The text and transmission of a Late Latin medical book*. London: Society for the Promotion of Roman Studies, 2006.

Opsomer, Carmelia. *Index de la pharmacopée du Ier au Xe siècle*, 2 vols. Hildesheim, Zürich, and New York, NY: Olms-Weidmann, 1989.

Pormann, Peter E. "Paulos of Aigina (*ca* 630 – 670 CE?)." In Paul T. Keyser and Georgia L. Irby-Massie (Eds.), *The encyclopedia of ancient natural scientists*. 625. London and New York, NY: Routledge, 2008.

Scarborough, John. "Philagrios of Ēpeiros (300 – 340 CE)." In Paul T. Keyser and Georgia L. Irby-Massie (Eds.), *The encyclopedia of ancient natural scientists*. 643-644. London and New York, NY: Routledge, 2008.

Zipser, Barbara. "Die *Therapeutica* des Alexander Trallianus: Ein medizinisches Handbuch und seine Überlieferung." In Rosa Marie Piccione and Matthias Perkams (Eds.), *Selecta Colligere, II. Beiträge zur Methodik des Sammelns von Texten in der Spätantike und in Byzanz (Collana Hellenika)*. 211-234. Alessandria: Edizioni dell'Orso, 2005.

Appendix 1

Manuscripts containing the Latin Alexander[88]

Complete copies

P1 Paris, *BN lat.* 9332 (early 9th cent.)
M Montecassino, *Archivio della Badia* 97 (early 10th cent.)
A Angers, *Bibl. mun.* 457 (11th cent.)
O Orléans, *Bibl. mun.* 283 (end 11th cent.)
D Durham, *Cathedral C.* 4. 11 (end 12th cent.)
G1 Glasgow, *University Library Hunter* 435 (12th-13th cent.)
Mu Munich, *BSB Clm* 344 (12th-13th cent.)
Ox Oxford, *Pembroke College* 8 (12th-13th cent.)
C Cambridge, *Gonville & Caius College* 400 (early 13th cent.)
Ge Geneva, *Bibl. publ. et univ.* 78 (13th cent.)
Ma Madrid, *BN* 1049 (13th cent.)
P2 Paris, *BNF lat.* 6881 (13th cent.)
P3 Paris, *BNF lat.* 6882 (13th cent.)
L2 London, *BL Royal* 12. B. XVI (late 13th cent.)
B Brussels, *KBR* 10869 (14th cent.)
G2 Glasgow, *University Library General* 1228 (second half 15th cent.)
L1 London, *BL Harley* 4914 (16th cent.)

Complete copies not seen by Langslow (before 2006)

Oxford, *Bodl.* 524 (12th cent)
Vatican City, *BAV Pal. lat.* 1209 (13th cent.)

Lost copies

Ch Chartres, *Bibl. mun.* 342 (12th cent.) – 'surviving only in a few photographs'
[**Metz** Metz, *Bibl. de la Ville ms.* 278 (early 13th cent.) – 'no reproductions of, or studies bearing on it are known' [89]

---

88 Langslow, *The Latin Alexander Trallianus...*, 38
89 Langslow, *The Latin Alexander Trallianus...*, 52-3 and n. 48

Appendix 2

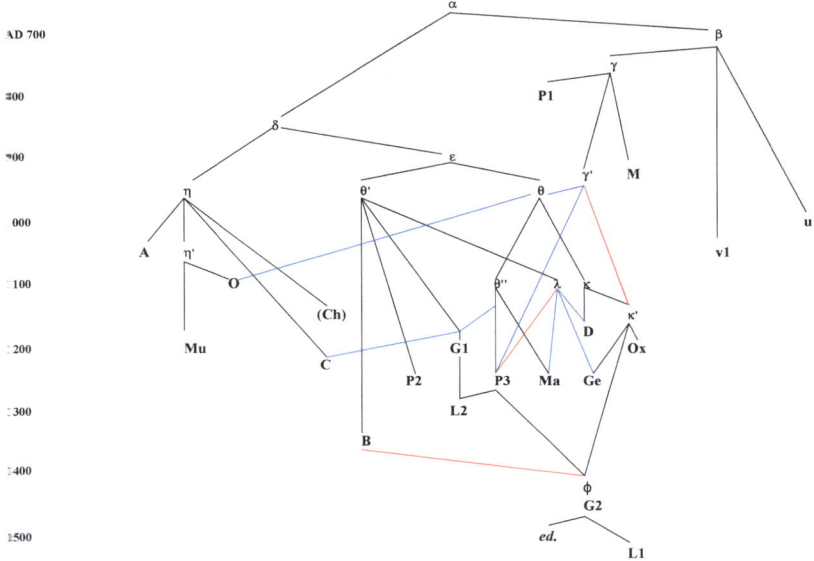

Figure 1. Stemma showing the relations between the mainstream manuscripts of the Latin
A.exander (and v1 and u of the secondary tradition). (Probable or certain use of an accessory model is
indicated in [blue], possible but uncertain use in [red]. The dating of lost copies is approximate only.).
Langslow, *The Latin Alexander Trallianus...*, Plate XII. Stemma reproduced with the kind permission of
David Langslow.

Appendix 3

Philumenus[90] (Transcript A, 1510, accessed from *Simon Online* 10.03.12, unless stated otherwise)

Acantis egyptia (Transcript A, 1510, last accessed 12.03.12)

A   **Acantis egyptia** *invenitur in practica Alexandri in confectione collirii ad tingenda leucemata puto quod sit idem quod achantis arabica.*

B   **Achantis egiptiaca** [*sic*] *inuenitur in pratica* [*sic*] *Ale. in confectione colirii* [*sic*] *ad tingenda leucomata puto quod sit idem quod achantis ara.*

2.79 *De reumate ventris Filominis* [*sic*] (Lyons 1504, 47r-48v)
48r: **acantis**[91] **egiptiace** [*sic*][92]
2.80 *De dissinteria reumatica* (Lyons 1504, 48v-49r)
48v: **achantem**[93] **egyptiam**[94]
2.98 *Enema ad dissintericos et dolores nimios vel inflammationes* (Lyons 1504, 51v-52r)
52r: **achanthos**[95] **egyptie**[96]
[Philagrius] 2.123 *De fomentationibus* (Lyons 1504, 55r-55v)
55v: **egyptie**[97] **acautis** [*sic*][98]

Epythyma elidion

A   **Epythyma elidion** *Alex. ca. de reumate ventris.*

B   **Epithima clidion** [*sic*] *Alex. capitulo de reumate uentris.*

2.79 *De reumate ventris Filominis* [*sic*] (Lyons 1504, 47r-48v)
47v: ... **Epithima dydyon**[99] [*sic*] *hoc modo conficitur.* ...

---

90 2.79-103: Lyons 1504, 47r-53r.
91 + gloss 'l': '*id est spine albe.*' (48r).
92 Cf. Mihăileanu, *Fragmentele latine...*, 110.7: *acantis aegyptias* [+ variants]; cf. Puschmann, *Nachträge zu Alexander Trallianus...*, 24: *acanthi Aegyptiacae* [no variants].
93 + gloss 'c': '*id est spinam al(_)s.*' (48v).
94 Cf. Mihăileanu, *Fragmentele latine...*, 116.10: *acantem egyptiam* [+ variants]; cf. Puschmann, *Nachträge zu Alexander Trallianus...*, 32: *acanthum Aegyptiacam* [no variants].
95 + gloss 'z': '*id est spine albe.*' (52r).
96 Cf. Mihăileanu, *Fragmentele latine...*, 139.11: *acantis egyptias* [+ variants]; cf. Puschmann, *Nachträge zu Alexander Trallianus...*, 62: *acanthi Aegyptiae* [no variants].
97 + gloss 'm': '*id est spine albe.*' (55v).
98 Cf. Mihăileanu, *Fragmentele latine...*, 165.2: *aegyptiae acantis* [+ variants]; cf. Puschmann, *Nachträge zu Alexander Trallianus...*, 96: *Aegyptiae acanthi* [no variants].
99 Cf. Mihăileanu, *Fragmentele latine...*, 108.4: *Epitima clidion* [+ variants]; cf. Puschmann, *Nachträge zu Alexander Trallianus...*, 22): *Epithema clidion* [no variants].

Ciliaca

A   **Ciliaca** *passio est fluxus ventris vitio stomachi nam .g. kiliam ventrem vocant ut in passionario suo ca. et est kilia fundus stomachi proprie. Item Alex. fit aut ex indigestione ventris defecti, liber de doctrina greca kilia alvus uterus venter.*

B   **Ciliaca** *passio est fluxus uentris uitio sto(_)a. nam gre. kiliam uentrem uocant ut in pasionario [sic] suo ca. et est kilia fundus sto(_)a. proprie. Item Alexan. fit autem ex indigestione uentris defecti: liber de doctrina gr(_). kilia koria aluus uter [sic] uenter.*

2.99 *De ciliacis Philomini* (Lyons 1504, 52r-52v)
[C]iliace[100] *passiones et indigestiones ex indigestione [sic] ipsius ventris fiunt eo quod non p(otes)t ex ipsa defectione ministrare corpori nutrimentum. ...*[101]

Embalmata (Transcript A, 1510, last accessed 12.03.12)

A   **Embalmata** *Alexan. ca. de medicinis ad frigidum stomachum, item de reumatismo ventris sunt intinctiones seu salsamenta in quibus morselli intinguntur.*
Embasmata **AC** | *Embalmata* **B e** | *iunctiones* **A** | *intinctiones* **B e** | *inunctiones* **C**

[Not 'Philumenus section'] **2.46** *Ad frigidum stomachum embalmata*[102] (Lyons 1504, 40v) [ms. **A** = *inbamata*]
40v: **[E]mbalmata** ... [for Greek ἔμβαμμα [sic]][103]

2.79 *De reumate ventris Filominis* [sic] (Lyons 1504, 47r-48v)
48r: *Item* **embalmata**[104] [105] [ms. **A** = *bamata*] *hoc modo ad hoc conficiuntur. Cimino cum salis modico et aceto oleo confecto intingitur quod edendum est.*

48v: *Potest autem iuuare et scorpio piscis assatus et cum cimini praedicti* **embalmate**[106] [107] *datus et ostree in suis testis assate et sumpte.*

---

100 + gloss 'l': '*est fluxus ventris vitio stamachi [sic].*' (52r).
101 Cf. Mihăileanu, *Fragmentele latine...*, 140.20-141.1: '*Ciliacae passiones ex indigestione ipsius ventris fiunt eo, quod ipse defectum patitur et non potest ex ipsa [141] defectione ministrare corpori nutrimenta.*' [+ variants]. Cf. Puschmann, *Nachträge zu Alexander Trallianus...*, 64: '*Coeliacae passiones ex indigestione ipsius ventris fiunt eo quod non potest ex ipsa defectione ministrare corpori nutrimentum.*' [+ variants].
102 + gloss 'f': '*sunt intinctiones seu salsamenta in quibus morselli intinguntur. Ian(_).*' (40v).
103 Πρὸς κατεψυγμένον στόμαχον ἔμβαμμα - Puschmann, *Alexander von Tralles...*, II.305.27.
104 + gloss 'c': '*sunt intinctiones seu salse [sic] in quibus morselli intinguntur. ian(_).*' (48r).
105 Cf. Mihăileanu, *Fragmentele latine...*, 112.8: *embammata* [no variants]; cf. Puschmann, *Nachträge zu Alexander Trallianus...*, 26: *embammata* [no variants].
106 + gloss 'a': '*id est salsamente.*' (48v).
107 Cf. Mihăileanu, *Fragmentele latine...*, 112.15: *embammate* [no variants]; cf. Puschmann, *Nachträge zu Alexander Trallianus...*, 26: *embammate* [no variants]

Appendix 4

Philagrius[108] (All Transcript A, 1510, last accessed from *Simon Online* 10.03.12)

Acantis egyptia: please see Appendix 3, Philumenus

Arthomeli

A   **Arthomeli** .g. panis cum melle factus Alex. ca. de cathaplasmatibus ad splenem cum ergo cognoveris et cetera.

B   **Artomeli** gr(_). panis cum melle factus Ale. capitulo de cataplasmatibus ad splenem cum ergo cognoueris et cetera.

2.129 *De cathaplasmate faciendo* (Lyons 1504, 56r-56v)
... Sepius autem sicut nouisti **artomelli**[109][110] usi sumus cum aqua. ...

Cinarum

A   **Cinarum** .g. Alex. ca. de cura calide et humide distemperantie splenis.

B   **Cinaron** [sic] g(_). Alexan. ca. de cura ca. de. [sic] et hu[|]de distemperatione splenis.

2.109 *Curatio calide et humide distperantie* [sic] (Lyons 1504, 53v-[5]4r)
... Carnes autem recentes edulina **cunarum**[111][112] spondilis[113] asp(er)agus[114] brionia et salsamenta omnia. ...

Clindonas

A   **Clindonas** greci Alexander ca. de ventositate splenis, clidonas enim greci vocant quando agitatur aqua sicut in utre ita in ventre.

B   **Clidonas** [sic] g(_). Alexan. ca. de uentositate splenis clidonas [sic] enim gre. uocant quando agitatur aqua sicut in utre ita in uentre.

2.115 *De ventositate splenis* (Lyons 1504, [5]4r)
... **Chimodas** [sic] [ms. **A** = **Clidonas**][115] namque Greci dicunt quando agitatur sicut in utre aqua ita et in ventre. ...

---

108 2.104-50: Lyons 1504, 53r-59r.
109 + gloss '"g"': 'Artomelli grece panis cum melle factus. Ian(_).' (56r).
110 Cf. Masullo Rita, *Filagrio: Framenti* (Naples: Bibliopolis, 1999), 332.437: *artomeli* [+ variants]; cf. Mihăileanu, *Fragmentele latine...*, 170.24: *artomele* [+ variants, 170-1]; cf. Puschmann, *Nachträge zu Alexander Trallianus...*, 102: *artomelle* [+ n. 128: ἀρτόμελι].
111 + gloss 'o': 'id est anser.' (53v).
112 Cf. Masullo, *Filagrio...*, 316.93: *cinnara* [+ variants]; cf. Mihăileanu, *Fragmentele latine...*,152.10: *cinnara* [+ variants]; cf. Puschmann, *Nachträge zu Alexander Trallianus...*, 78: *cinara* [+ variants].
113 + gloss 'p': 'id est caro spondilium.' (53v).
114 + gloss 'q': 'id est sp(er)agus.' (53v).
115 Cf. Masullo, *Filagrio...*, 319.161: *Clidonas* [no variants]; cf. Mihăileanu *Fragmentele latine...*, 155.16: *Clidonas* [no variants]; cf. Puschmann, *Nachträge zu Alexander Trallianus...*, 84: *Clydonas* [no variants].

Epilata

A ***Epilata*** *.g. medicine laxative per os sumpte ut Alex. ca. de splene, nunc ergo dicendum et cetera, sunt maxime leves ut idem infra de epilatibus illa ergo danda et cetera.*

B ***Epilata*** *gr(_). medi(_)e laxati(_)e per os sumpte ut Alex. capitulo de splene nunc ergo dandum [sic] est et cetera. sunt maxime lenes [sic] ut idem infra de opilato(n)ibus [sic] illa igitur danda et cetera.*

2.121 *Curatio flegmonis in splene generati* **(Lyons 1504, 55r)**
[N]unc igitur dicendum est de inflammatione in splene generata. ... Alie quidem euacuationes sunt que per ventrem deponunt[116] *quas Greci* **epilatas**[117] *vocant que sunt in primis utende. ...*

2.122 De epilatibus[118 119]**(Lyons 1504, 55r)**
[E]pilata[120] *igitur danda sunt que euacuare solent per ventrem qui continentur humores post flobothomum: habebis enim in hiis exemplum sicut in quarto libro de podagricis scriptum est. Sunt enim* **epilata** *leuia medicamenta qualia sunt herba mercurialis et polipodium et gincus*[121] *et acalafis*[122] *semen et hiis similia.*

2.127 *De catartico aut apozimate vel inunctionibus* **(Lyons 1504, 56r)**
[C]um ergo meliorata fuerit passio mutanda sunt adiutoria et purgandus est venter de **epilatis**[123 124] *mitibus per os datis coctis in ptisanis / aut cum aqua danda sunt ad bibendum. ...*

2.134 *Curatio scyron splenis* **(Lyons 1504, 57r)**
... Tunc a nobis duobus aut tribus diebus **epilatis**[125 126] *catarticis purgatus est. ...*

2.137 *De sanguine tollendo* **(Lyons 1504, 57r-57v)**
... Postea autem cum bene resolutum esset splen de **epilatis**[127] *dedi catarticis et euacuaui vacantes humores per ventrem fortioribus medicamentis [57v] id est antidotis dyacolloquintidos yere ...*

---

116 + gloss 'e': '*id est euacuant.*' (55r).
117 Cf. Masullo, *Filagrio...,* 325.272: *epilata* [+ variant]; cf. Mihăileanu, *Fragmentele latine...,* 161.7): *epilata* [no variants]; cf. Puschmann, *Nachträge zu Alexander Trallianus...,* 92: *hypelata* [+ n. 73: ὑπήλατα].
118 + gloss 'h': '*id est medicine laxatiue per os sumpte* [sic]. *Ian(_).*' (55r).
119 Cf. Masullo, *Filagrio...,* 325.293: *epilatis* [+ variants]; cf. Mihăileanu, *Fragmentele latine...,* 162.13): *epilatis* [+ variants]; cf. Puschmann, *Nachträge zu Alexander Trallianus...,* 92: *hypelatis* [no variants].
120 Cf. Masullo, *Filagrio...,* 325.293: *Epilata* [no variants]; cf. Mihăileanu, *Fragmentele latine...,* 162.13: *Epilata* [no variants]; cf. Puschmann, *Nachträge zu Alexander Trallianus...,* 92: *Hypelata* [no variants].
121 + gloss 'i': '*gincus est crocus hortulanus. Ian(_).*' (55r).
122 + gloss 'k': '*id est urtice.*' (55r).
123 + gloss 'b': '*id est medicinis laxatiuis per os assumpis.* [sic]' (56r).
124 Cf. Masullo, *Filagrio...,* 330.386: *epilatis* [+ variants]; cf. Mihăileanu, *Fragmentele latine...,* 168.5): *epilatis* [no variants]; cf. Puschmann, *Nachträge zu Alexander Trallianus...,* 98: *hypelatis* [no variants].
125 + gloss 'd': '*id est medicinis laxatiuis per os sumptis.* [sic]' (57r).
126 Cf. Masullo, *Filagrio...,* 336.522: *epilatis* [no variants]; cf. Mihăileanu, *Fragmentele latine...,* 175.11: *epilatis* [no variants]; cf. Puschmann, *Nachträge zu Alexander Trallianus...,* 108: *hypelatis* [no variants].
127 Cf. Masullo, *Filagrio...,* 338.567: *epilatis* [no variants]; cf. Mihăileanu, *Fragmentele latine...,* 177.11: *epilatis* [no variants]; cf. Puschmann, *Nachträge zu Alexander Trallianus...,* 110-112: *hypelatis* [no variants].

Epythyma ypotirion

A   **Epythyma ypotirion** idem Alex. de splene.

B   **Epithima ypotirion** idem Alex. capitulo de splene.

2.145 **Epithima ypotirion**[128] (Lyons 1504, 58v)
[S]unt autem et alia epithimata[129] ad spleneticos et ydropicos que nominantur ypotirion[130]. ...

Eukrion

A   **Eukrion** Alex. de cura ventositatis splenis prassii **eucrion** et cetera.

B   **Eukrion** Alex. de cura uentositatis splenis prassii **eukrion** et cetera.

2.116 Curatio ventositatis (Lyons 1504, [5]4r-[5]4v)
[[5]4v] ... Sed et alia sunt qualis est herpillus et thimus et lauri cortex et origanum. Et calamentum siccum et viride et piper et ruthe semen / et maxime si siluestris sit et pencedanum[131] [sic] et maxime opos[132] ipsius et costum et cardamomum et prassium. et **eucrion**[133] [134] [ms. **A** = **ucrion**] et centaurea subtilis...

Omotribum oleum

A   **Omotribum oleum** Alex. ca. de cephalea, **omotribus oleum** inquit octobriscum et cetera. Idem in ca. de fomentis ad splenis inflationem. Item in ca. de linimentis ad podagram calidam, **oleo** inquit **omotribio** quod primo tempore fit et recipit folia olive ut sit amarum et cetera, Ga. vero .xi. de ingenio, oleum onfacinum, ab aliis vero **omotriuos** .i. ex acerbis olivis constructum et cetera.

B   **Omotribum oleum** Alex. ca. de cephalea **omotribum ol(eu)m** inquit .i. octobriscum et cetera idem in ca. de linimentis idem in c. de fomentatione ad splenis in fla(_)ationem idem in capitulo de linimentis ad podagram calidam **oll(e)o** [sic] inquit **omotribio** quod primo tempore fit et recipit folia oliue ut sit amarum et cetera. Gal(_) uero in io [sic] de ingenio sanitatis ol(eu)m onfaci(n)um [sic] ab aliis uero **omotrinos** [sic] .i. ex acerbis oliuis constructum et cetera.

---

128 Cf. Masullo, *Filagrio...*, 348.765: *Epitima ypotirion* [+ variants]; cf. Mihăileanu, *Fragmentele latine...*,186.1: *Epitima ypotirion* [+ variants]; cf. Puschmann, *Nachträge zu Alexander Trallianus...*, 120: *Epithema hypotherion* [no variants].
129 Cf. Masullo, *Filagrio...*, 348.766: *epitimata* [no variants]; cf. Mihăileanu, *Fragmentele latine...*,186.1: *epitimata* [no variants]; cf. Puschmann, *Nachträge zu Alexander Trallianus...*, 120: *epithemata* [no variants].
130 Cf. Masullo, *Filagrio...*, 348.766: *ypotirion* [+ variants]; cf. Mihăileanu, *Fragmentele latine...*,186.2: *ipoterion* [+ variants]; cf. Puschmann, *Nachträge zu Alexander Trallianus...*, 120: *hypotheria* [no variants].
131 + gloss 'm': 'id est feniculus porcinus.' ([5]4v).
132 + gloss 'n': 'id est succus.' ([5]4v).
133 + gloss 'o': 'eukrion per k scribit ianuensis allegans hunc passum. sed non exponit extimo quod sit eupatorium.' ([5]4v).
134 Cf. Masullo, *Filagrio...*, 321.197: *teucrion* [+ variants]; cf. Mihăileanu, *Fragmentele latine...*,157.11: *teucrion* [+ variants]; cf. Puschmann, *Nachträge zu Alexander Trallianus...*, 86: *teucrium* [no variants].

2.123 *De fomentationibus* (Lyons 1504, 55r-55v)
[55v] ... *Quod si calor sit mittendum est oleum* **omotribe**[135][136] *et rosa.* ...

[Not 'Philagrius section'] 2.155 *De ydrope asclite et tympanite* (Lyons 1504, 68v)
... *Nihilominus autem faciende sunt fricationes cum sale et oleo* **omotribro**[137] [*sic*] [for Greek ὠμοτριβοῦς[138]] *et sicionio*[139] *et ciprino.* ...

[Not 'Philagrius section', section on gout] 2.245 *De amplastris* (76r-76v)
[76v] ... *Quod si oleum roseum non adest cum oleo* **omotrible** [*sic*] [for Greek **ὠμοτριβές**[140]] *id est amaro quod primo tempore fit et recipit folia oliue ut sit amarum utilissimum est.* ...

[Not 'Philagrius section'] 1.40 *Curatio cephalargicorum* (Lyons 1504, 6r-6v)
... *oportet adhibere et fomentationes cum altea vel oleo aut herbis in aqua coctis non satis calidis sed et robur habentibus ut confortare valeant caput quale est* **omotribem** [6v] *id est* **octobrinum** [ms. **A** = **octobrisicum**] [for Greek **ὠμοτριβές**[141]] *oleum .s. amarum quod primo tempore fit et accipit* [*sic*] *folia oliue ut sit amarum. utilissimum enim est* ...

Pegmata

A   **Pegmata** *.g. Alex. ca. de dieta inflationis splenis li. de doctrina .g. pegmata vel pigmata vel* · *pigmenta.*

B   **Peginata** [*sic*] *gr*(_). *Alex. ca. de dieta inflationis splenis liber de doctrina gr*(_) *peginata* [*sic*] *pigmata pigmenta:* [*sic*]

2.105 *Signa frigide distemperantie splenis* (Lyons 1504, 53r)
... *Qualia sunt aqua frigida ostrea sterilis*[142] *caro porcina pomorum copia accepta et diuersa* **poma** [ms. **A** = **pimmata**][143] *et maxime in estate accepta.* ...

---

135 + gloss 'b': *'id est oleum oliuarum quod primo tempore fit et recipit folia oliue ut sit cmarum. Ianuensis.'* (55v).
136 Cf. Masullo, *Filagrio...*, 326.313: omotribe [+ variants]; cf. Mihăileanu, *Fragmentele latine...*,164.1: omotribe [+ variants]; cf. Puschmann, *Nachträge zu Alexander Trallianus...*, 94: cmotribes [+ n. 83: ὠμοτριβές].
137 + gloss 'e': *'id est oleum oliuarum quod primo tempore fit et recipit folia oliue ut magis sit amarum.'* (68v).
138 Puschmann, *Alexander von Tralles...*, II.449.33.
139 + gloss 'f': *'id est de radice cucumeris agrestis.'* (68v).
140 Puschmann, *Alexander von Tralles...*, II.517.20.
141 Puschmann, *Alexander von Tralles...*, I.491.1
142 + gloss 'r': *'id est omasa.'* (53r).
143 Cf. Masullo, *Filagrio...*, 312.15: pemmata [+ variants]; cf. Mihăileanu, *Fragmentele latine...*,148.16: pemmata [+ variants]; cf. Puschmann, *Nachträge zu Alexander Trallianus...*, 74: pemmata [+ variants].

Sisti

A
Sisti *etiam aliquando pro eodem alumine reperitur et etiam pro arsenico nam utrumque* **scissile** *est ut Alex. confectione ethionica ad splenem.*

B
Sisti *etiam aliquando pro eodem alu(m)i(n)e reperitur et etiam pro arsenico nam utrumque* **scisille** *[sic] est ut Alex. in conf(e)c(ti)one epithonica [sic] ad splenem.*

2.141 *Confectio epithimatis atonotici*[144] *ad splen [sic] confortandum* (**Lyons 1504, 58r**)
[M]edicamen quod supra diximus de arsenico et stipterea et confortatio ad splenem seu splenis athomam[145] *quam superposui homini illi quem sepius memorauimus. quod recipit ... arsenici* **sciscis**[146] [147] *... auripigmenti* **scissilis**[148] *... stipteree* [**ms. A** = *stipteria* **scistis**][149] *...*

---

144 + gloss 'b': '*id est confortatiui seu roboratiui.*' (58r).
145 + gloss 'c': '*debilitatem. lan(_).*' (58r).
146 + gloss 'e': '*a loco.*' (58r).
147 Cf. Cf. Masullo, *Filagrio...*, 344.692: *scisto* [+ variants]; cf. Mihăileanu, *Fragmentele latine...*, 181.18: *scisto* [+ variants]; cf. Puschmann, *Nachträge zu Alexander Trallianus...*, 116: *scissi* [no variants].
148 Cf. Masullo, *Filagrio...*, 344.693: *scissili* [+ variants]; cf. Mihăileanu, *Fragmentele latine...*, 181.19): *scissili* [+ variants]; cf. Puschmann, *Nachträge zu Alexander Trallianus...*, 116: omitted, and no variants.
149 Cf. Masullo, *Filagrio...*, 344.693: *scistis* [+ variants]; cf. Mihăileanu, *Fragmentele latine...*, 181.19-182.1: *stipteria scistis* [+ variants]; cf. Puschmann, *Nachträge zu Alexander Trallianus...*, 116: *stypteriae scissilis* [no variants].

Edited by **Barbara Zipser**

Caroline Petit

Galen's Pharmacological Concepts and Terminology in Simon of Genoa's *Clavis sanationis*

Among the many works on plants from antiquity and the middle ages that have come down to us, Galen's treatise *Simple Medicines*, in eleven books,[1] stands out not only because of its length (about a thousand pages in the standard Kühn edition), but also because it lays special emphasis on the properties of plants, animals, and minerals used as simple medicines. Instead of merely describing s mples, as many of his predecessors and followers did, Galen devoted five books out of eleven to defining the correct method in using drugs. Books VI-XI then examine the *materia medica* in alphabetical order, highlighting the properties of each substance, instead of providing a detailed description and a full list of synonyms. In the Islamic world, *Simple medicines* was widely used and its method for classifying medicines according to their power and action was reinforced and systematized. The works of Avicenna, Al-Jazzar, and Al-Razi, to mention but a few, show evidence of Galen's influence in this respect.[2] As Simon of Genoa relied heavily on Islamic medical works and their translations, I had initially anticipated to find at least indirect evidence of Galenic ideas on pharmacology in the *Clavis Sanationis*; it soon appeared that Simon used directly several Galenic works, including the treatise *Simple Medicines*. Simon, however, used Galen's treatise but paid little attention to Galen's method. In fact, Simon's debt to Galen is not as overwhelming as one could be tempted to believe: I found a number of words quoted from Galen, but not the words I expected. I was hoping to find evidence of Galenic methodology in the use of drugs; instead I found considerations on the naming of plants, where Galen is only one of the many sources used by Simon. Therefore Galen's place in the *Clavis Sanationis* is not as prominent as I had hoped. The aim of this paper is to try and explain why, by reviewing Simon's Galenic sources, and in turn to examine whether the *Clavis sanationis* is of any use for the edition of Galen's text.

---

[1] *De simpl. med. fac. ac. temp.*, in *Claudii Galeni Opera Omnia (1821-1833)*, vol. XI, 379-XII, 372.

[2] Peter E. Pormann, "The Formation of the Arabic Pharmacology Between Tradition and Innovation", in *Annals of Science* 68-4 (2011): 493-515.

Reading through the *Clavis Sanationis'* entries, it quickly occurred to me that Simon was particularly interested in the names and descriptions of plants more than their healing properties. Whenever possible, he provides synonyms and tells us of the many ways in which a plant can be named according to authors and places. Indeed, Simon's preface is very clear that linguistic variation around the names of the *materia medica* is an important factor of the transmission of texts, and one of the main difficulties for the readers and users of such books.[3] For the sake of both clarity and the history of medicine, Simon provided as much information as he could, even when a particular name did not seem to be in use any more: for he feared that some technical terms might be lost forever. This explains in great part why Simon's work, in theory at least, is so precious to historians of pharmacy and pharmacology: the *Clavis sanationis* may in some cases contain evidence of lost manuscripts, or of earlier recensions of medical treatises that we know. It also shows how the pharmacological texts of the past were read, understood, and used for the sake of therapeutics or simply for the sake of increasing knowledge. In the case of Galen, however, the particular case of the treatise on *Simple medicines* shows that Simon could not make much use of this text, and that the *Clavis*, in turn, has little to tell us about the textual history and for the edition of the text.

Galenic Sources in Simon's *Clavis*:

There is no evidence that Simon had access to Galen's works in the Greek original. Rather, it seems that he had to rely on a variety of Latin translations; those were made either from a Greek original or from its Arabic translation. In addition, the material is a curious mix of authentic and spurious works; some were transmitted in Latin as early as late antiquity, through Latin translations that were probably made in Italy, although not all can be traced back to the famous

---

3 Simon, *Clavis*, Praef.: *Sunt medicinarum simplicium ciborum ve multa peregrina vocabula: quorum quedam a greca: quedam vero ab arabica lingua deducta sunt. Nonulla et quamquam latina varietate idiomatum dubia: ad quorum omnium agnitionem non opus est assertione facili sed deliberato iudicio: ne ut neglectu medico grave et irreparabile occurat dispendium.* There are many foreign terms for simple medicines and foodstuffs. Some of these are derived from the Greek language, some from the Arabic language. A few words are also unclear in the Latin language. To recognise all of these, we do not need easy claims, but reasoned judgement, so that a physician does not meet grave and irreparable damage through negligence.

school of Ravenna – such is the case, however, of the treatise *Ad Glauconem* in two books, mentioned and quoted several times by Simon.[4]

In the following, I list Galenic works mentioned in the preface, and works mentioned elsewhere in the text. Naturally, this survey is based on partial research in the *Clavis* and more titles could eventually appear. The difficulty lies in Simon's method of quotation: usually, Galen appears simply as 'Gal.', 'Gali.' or even 'G.' The latter makes searching the online edition of the *Clavis* slightly difficult, as the same abbreviation could be used for various other words. The same applies to work titles, which are not quoted consistently throughout the *Clavis*. Another problem is that Simon may not have cited his sources systematically; thus quotations of Galen could lie undetected in the text. But this is unlikely, given his usually scrupulous manner in referencing the material he used. Simon also specifies in the preface that some works, such as the *Ad Glauconem*, were not of great use to him when composing the *Clavis sanationis*. Thus it is certainly possible that he doesn't quote or mention works that he did not believe to be valuable.

Galenic Works Explicitly Mentioned in the *Clavis sanationis*:

N B. : for each work I specify the language I surmise the text was translated from, whether Simon is explicit or not on this matter; I also provide examples from Simon's quotations to support each hypothesis.

- in the preface § 4:

> *ad Glauconem (*'for Glaucon'), in two books, one on fevers, one on abscesses (late antique Latin translation from the Greek)
> *de alimentis ('on food', *De alim. facultatibus*? *De alimentis* is no standard title[5]), translated from the Greek (see for ex. *arkeutidas*) – see below *de cibis*

---

4 About the rich diffusion of this fundamental Galenic work, see for example Ivan Garofalo, "La traduzione araba dei compendi alessandrini delle opere del canone di Galeno. Il compendio dell'Ad Glauconem." *Medicina nei Secoli N.S.* 6 (1994): 329– 348; Keith Dickson, *Stephanus the philosopher and physician: commentary on Galen's* Therapeutics to Glaucon. *Introd., Greek text with critical apparatus and index of sources, English transl., notes.* (Leiden: Brill, 1998); Bengt Löfstedt, "Zum Lateinischen Kommentar von Galens Ad Glaucone," in Joszef Herman (Ed.) *Latin vulgaire – latin tardif. Actes du Ier Colloque international sur le latin vulgaire et tardif (Pécs, 2–5 septembre 1985)*, (Tübingen: Niemeyer, 1987), 145–151.
5 See Gerhard Fichtner, *Corpus Galenicum. Ein Verzeichnis der galenischen und pseudo-galenischen Schriften*, Tübingen, accessible online on the website of the *Corpus Medicorum Graecorum* in Berlin http://cmg.bbaw.de/online-publications/Galen-Bibliographie_2012_08_28.pdf , 2011.

Arkeutidas vocant grece fructum iuniperi, secundum Gali. in liber de alimentis.
Arkeutidas they call in Greek the fruit of juniper trees, according to Galen in his book on food.
*liber sextus de simplicibus medicinis ('the sixth book on simple medicines'), translated from the Arabic (see below)
*ad Paternianum ('for Paternianus', ps. Gal), translated from the Greek.

- elsewhere:

*de ingenio sanitatis ('on the method of healing', =De Methodo Medendi), translated from the Greek, see for example[6]:
Calastica [...] exponitur tamen in libro Gali. de ingenio sanitatis de greco translato quod est remissiva. [...] Calastica [...] is also furthering remission, as it is outlined in Galen's book *on the method of healing*, in the translation from the Greek.
*de cibis ('on food', this is the standard title of *De alim. fac.* in Latin), translated from the Greek, see for example:
Candarusium [...] D. vero vocat ipsum condros: et sic vocatur grece et in libro de cibis Gali. ca. proprium scribit [...]. Candarusium [...] but Dioscorides calls it *condros*: and it is called thus in Greek, and Galen writes a dedicated chapter on it in the book *on food*.
*Condros [...] Gal. in li. de alimentis genus frumenti est condros sufficienter nutritivum viscosum habens chimum [...]*Condros [...] Galen says in the book *on food* that condros is a type of cereal, that is sufficiently nutritious and has a sticky juice.
* de virtutibus naturalibus ('on natural faculties'), translated from the Greek, see for example:
Emagogum sanguis eductivum Gal. in li. de virtutibus naturalibus. Emagogum is an agent that expels blood, Galen in the book *on natural faculties*.
*de secretis Galieni ('Galen's book on secrets', = *liber secretorum ad Monteum*)

Translated from the Arabic, as shown by the following examples (I have compared Simon's text with an early printed edition from 1550 systematically):

Ciminum carmenum exponitur in secretis .G. in medicina quam fecit Herodi ad stomachum quod est siseleos [...] Ciminum carmenum is described in Galen's book *on secrets* in a medicine which he attributes to Herodes for the stomach, that is *siselos* [...][7]

---

6 The quotations from the *Clavis* follow the transcription on the *Simon Online* website. Meaningful variant readings are discussed in footnotes.
7 Cf. Lyon 1550 edition, tom. IV, 1145-46. *cymini*

Felenia Gal. in secretis in confectione quadam ad debilitatem anime vide si est idem quod felemenusch.[8] *Felenia*, Galen in the book *on secrets* in a recipe for the weakness of the soul, see whether it is the same as *felemenusch*.[9]

Rubie [...] *in secretis vero Gal. in sief conservatio visus rubien invenitur. Rubie* [...] but in Galen's book *on secrets* in *sief* one can find that *rubien* is an agent that preserves vision.[10]

Birenum vas est de lapide .s. lebes sustinens ignem, in secretis G. in descriptione rob de fructibus. Birenum is a vessel made of stone such as a bowl for fire, in Galen's book *on secrets* it appears in the description of rob made from fruits.[11]

Massacumia [...] *vel potius Gal. in secretis unde ipsum extrahit exponunt eum quod est aqua vitri quod quidem ignoro quid sit* [...][12] *Massacumia* [...] but more likely is here Galen in his book *on secrets* on where he extracts it from: 'they explain that it is glass water'. But I don't know what it is.[13]

Some of the Galenic works used and cited by Simon of Genoa belong to the famous 'Alexandrian Canon'[14], such as the *Therapeutic method* and the *Natural faculties*; others are spurious texts which became more or less popular in the middle ages, such as the treatise preserved only in Latin and titled *Ad Faternianum*, sometimes called *Alfabetum Galieni*. Carmelia Opsomer has devoted a substantial study to that text, its sources, and its textual history, in the wider context of ancient pharmacological works transmitted in the Middle Ages

---

8 *Felemenusch* AC | *felemeli vel felemeki* vel *fememieh* vel *felememise* B | *felelemisch* f | *felemelum* vel *felememisch* e. Witnesses B fe form one distinct group of the transmission. Since only part of this group contains several more synonyms, these most likely reflect scholia by a later hand, which were added at some point in the B branch, but only incorporated into the main text by some scribes.

9 Cf. Lyon ed. 1550, 1147 *felinia felifelias, id est, agni casti*.

10 Lyon ed. 1550, 1142 *modus sief*.

11 Cf. Lyon ed. 1550, 1145 *bireno scilicet lebete*.

12 *Aqua vitri* AC e | *aqua vitri aqua vasorum vitri* B | *aqua vitri et aqua vasorum vitri* f. Again, as in the footnote above, only parts of the B ef branch transmit a synonym, which indicates that this goes back to a scholion.

13 Cf. Lyon ed. 1550, 1142 *massae cumiae*.

14 Vivian Nutton, "Medicine in Late Antiquity and the Early Middle Ages," in Lawrence I. Conrad et al. (Eds.), *The Western Medical Tradition*. Cambridge: Cambridge University Press, 1995, reprint 2007, 81.

in the West.[15] The presence of genuinely Galenic material in that very popular text remains to be properly assessed.

Simon is often very clear that he used a translation from the Arabic or from the Greek; even when he is not explicit, it is relatively easy to spot a translation made from either language, as I hope the examples above make clear for each of the 'Galenic' works mentioned by Simon.

Due to variation in works' titles in the medieval period, the book called *De secretis Galieni* ('Galen's book on secrets'), translated from the Arabic, could have been one of two works, either the *Liber secretorum ad Monteum* ('The book on secrets for Monteus', in the form of a letter), or the *De secretis virorum/ mulierorum* ('On the secrets of men/women').[16] But a quick comparison between the passages cited by Simon and one of the editions of the *Liber secretorum ad Monteum* shows that Simon used that work, and not the other.

What source did Simon exactly use for each of these texts is of course difficult to state: it would be necessary to know of the textual transmission of each text in detail. Sometimes, as in the case of the treatise *Natural faculties*, there is a single mention of the text, and it makes it virtually impossible to make an attempted reconstitution of Simon's source. The relative lack of manuscripts transmitting Galenic works around the thirteenth century makes this task impossible. In the case of Galen's treatise on *Simple medicines*, it is particularly clear that Simon had little at hand when he wrote the *Clavis*. A simple hypothesis, however, is that he may have had access to a collection of Galenic works in Latin, perhaps bound with yet other texts by different authors. For some of the works he barely quotes (once or twice), he may even have used an intermediary source. At any rate, Galen's *Simple medicines* provide an interesting, if frustrating, case study.

Galen's Eleven Books *On simple medicines* and Simon's *Clavis sanationis*

The examples presented below show that Simon used exclusively a Latin translation of that text, and that it was made from the Arabic. For various reasons, it is very unlikely that he also viewed Greek manuscripts.

---

15 Carmelia Opsomer-Halleux, "Un herbier médicinal du haut moyen-âge: l'*alfabetum galieni*", *History and Philosophy of the Life Sciences* 4 (1982): 65-97. For an English translation see also Everett, *The Alphabet of Galen. Pharmacy from Antiquity to the Middle Ages*, (Toronto: University of Toronto Press, 2011).

16 On which see Fichtner, *Corpus Galenicum*.

The Improbable Greek Manuscript.

In principle, Simon could have accessed Greek manuscripts in Italy. Some of Galen's books were produced in Southern Italy even before Simon's lifetime[17]. But in the case of Galen's *Simple medicines*, this hypothesis is difficult to back up. The Greek manuscript material is frustrating, because it is either in a poor condition, or fragmentary, or late and corrupt.[18] Nevertheless, we do have some relatively old manuscripts (the oldest dating from the tenth century). Their current condition and their usefulness for the edition vary. At any rate, they are likely to have remained in Constantinople from their creation in the tenth to fourteenth century until the fifteenth century, when they were re-used and sometimes restored by the likes of Demetrios Angelos and *then* brought to Italy. Such is the pattern for the manuscripts concerning the first part of the text, Books I-V: they have their origins in Constantinople.[19] But Books I-V on the one hand, and VI-XI on the other hand, have had a different fate. Each half of the text was transmitted in different manuscripts; the existence of copies of the full text is due to relatively late (fifteenth century) combination of manuscripts of both sections of the text. This bipartition of the Greek tradition is in part reflected in the indirect tradition, especially in Latin. Concerning the Greek manuscripts that are of interest for the edition of the second part of *Simple medicines*, the *Palatinus gr.* 31, for example, deserves further study: it is perhaps older than the fourteenth century date given by the catalogue, and I cannot prove at present that it never was in Italy, as it would require extensive research and direct

---

17 On this controversial topic, see for example Jean Irigoin, "La tradition de l'*Ars medica* de Galien dans l'Italie meridionale." *Bollettino della Badia graeca di Grottaferrata* N.S. 4 (1991): 5, 85-91; Anna Maria Ieraci Bio, "La trasmissione della letteratura medica greca nell'Italia meridionale fra X e XV secolo." In Antonio Garzya (Ed.), *Contributi alla cultura Greca nell'Italia meridionale*, (Naples: Bibliopolis, 1989), 133-255 and Guglielmo Cavallo, "La trasmissione scritta della cultura greca antica in Calabria e in Sicilia tra i secoli X e XV: Consistenza, tipologia, fruizione." *Scrittura e Civiltà* 4 (1980): 157-245.

18 About the textual transmission of Galen's XI books on *Simple medicines*, see Caroline Petit "La tradition manuscrite du traité des Simples de Galien. *Editio princeps* et traduction annotée des chapitres 1 a 3 du livre I." in Véronique Boudon-Millot, Jacques Jouanna, Antonio Garzya, Amneris Roselli (Eds.), *Histoire de la tradition et édition des médecins grecs - Storia della tradizione e edizione dei medici greci*, (Napoli: D'Auria, 2010), 143-165 and "Théorie et pratique: connaissance et diffusion du traite des *Simples* de Galien au Moyen Age." in Arsenio Ferraces Rodriguez (Ed.), *Fito-zooterapia antigua y altomedieval: textos y doctrinas*, (A Coruna: Univ. da Coruna, Servizo de Publicacions, 2009), 79-95.

19 When I worked on the textual transmission of Galen's *Simple medicines* several years ago, I focussed my attention on this first part of the text and did less research on books VI-XI, which are precisely the books that Simon may have used.

inspection of the manuscript.[20] Therefore we cannot rule out the possibility of a Greek manuscript accessed by Simon of Genoa, but Simon himself does not give a hint of that, and I think that what we know of the manuscript tradition makes it difficult to give credit to this hypothesis.

I do not intend to describe at length the Greek tradition but, because it is of relevance later, I want to emphasize that, due to the dimensions of the text, too big perhaps for a single codex, the manuscripts each only have half of the text, either Books I-V or Books VI-XI, with the single exception of a fragmentary manuscript now in Milan, which has bits and pieces of Books V to IX and was perhaps our only old manuscript containing the entire text.[21] This bipartition had consequences for the history of the text: in the first place, the two parts of the treatise, the theoretical and the practical, are transmitted by different manuscripts and have two distinct textual histories. They were presumably not read together, or by the same people. The complete texts printed in the sixteenth century arise from reconstitutions made in the fifteenth to sixteenth century, when the two parts of the text were eventually – and artificially – brought together from separate manuscripts.

Later on, the various translation movements in the East and in the West were influenced by this bipartition – in the medieval West, in particular, the Latin manuscripts usually display either Part I (Book I-V), or Part II (Books VI-XI). When the two parts appear together in a manuscript, it is not an indication that they belong to the same translation. Moreover, individual books may reflect several different translations, and the situation is not as clear as we might wish, as I will explain shortly. It is commonplace to distinguish between old, twelfth century translations made from the Arabic or, more rarely, from the Greek; and the second, bigger wave of translations in the fourteenth century, with a majority of Latin versions made from the Greek, for example by Niccolò da Reggio. This schematic approach does not do justice to the complexity of the transmission of all Galenic works, but in the case of Galen's treatise on *Simple medicines*, it works relatively well.[22]

---

20 There is no scholarship on this manuscript. The style of the handwriting, to me, looks similar to that of George Galesiotes; but this old-fashioned style remained popular for decades, which makes perilous any attempt at giving a secure date. The paper is oriental, hence bears no filigranes that would help locate the making of this manuscript in time and place.

21 Milan, *Ambr. A 81 inf. (gr. 802)*.

22 My study of the Latin tradition of Galen's *Simple medicines*, will appear in the proceedings of the conference organised by S. Fortuna on the Latin translations of Galen's works (Ancona, 31 May-1 June 2012).

The Latin Translation(s).

The examples that I append clearly show that Simon's explicit quotations from Galen's text come from a Latin translation made from a manuscript in Arabic. At the beginning of each of the entries in the Latin translation of Book VI, as it appears in two different sources, a printed edition of 1490 (the famous two-volume complete edition curated by Diomedes Bonardus, Venice) and a fourteenth century Latin manuscript (Vatican, *BAV Pal. lat.* 1094), the text has an Arabic name (spelled in Latin characters) next to the Latin one. The printed edition, however, has chapter numbers and headings that are not found in the *Pal. lat.* 1094; there are also some slight orthographic differences. I presume that the editor used a different manuscript, not the *Pal. lat.* 1094, but it is the only one that I was able to check for the purpose of this study.[23] Most of the time, it is in fact inaccurate to talk of 'quotations' from Galen's text: indeed, Simon only mentions occurrences of plant names as found in Galen's text, or abruptly summarizes one of its brief chapters. Hence my study merely consists in identifying the relevant passages in the Latin translation ascribed to Gerard of Cremona, both in the 1490 edition and in ms. *Pal. lat.* 1094. Wherever possible, I also mention the Arabic word that corresponds to the Latin term, as provided by M. Ullmann in his Greco-Arabic dictionary.[24] On some occasions, the two translations of Book VI (one ascribed to Hunain, one by Al-Bitriq) studied by Ullmann differ, but the Latin word usually shows which model was used, and it is most certainly Hunain's.

Quotations from Galen's *Simple medicines*, Book VI:

(1) *Berengesif* [...] *veritas est quod berengesif est artemisia, nam in .vi. de simplici medicina G. exponit quod .g. dicitur artemisia, poro si conparas ca. eius cum ca. de artemisia apud D. videbis quod idem dicunt* [...] *Berengesif* [...] the truth is that *berengesif* is artemisia, for Galen writes in the sixth book of *Simple Medicines* that it is called artemisia in Greek, moreover, if you compare his chapter with the chapter on artemisia in Dioscoride, you will see that they say the same [...]
Gal. lat. 1490 *belengesif,* cap. 58 *De artemisia*
Pal. lat. 1094 f. 557r: *belengresif – arthemesia*
Arabic: cf. Ullmann, p. 136 (Hunain: *belengresif;* Al-Bitriq: *artemisia*)

23 Whenever the *Pal. lat.* 1094 reading is not mentioned, it means that I could not read the (poor) photocopies at my disposal properly.
24 Manfred Ullmann, *Wörterbuch zu den griechisch-arabischen Übersetzungen des neunten Jahrhunderts,* (Wiesbaden: Harrassovitz, 2002).

(2) *Achavē* [...] *ut in .vi. G. de simplicibus medicinis ubi alachoen scribitur* [...] *Achavē* [...] as in the sixth book of Galen's *Simple medicines* where he writes *alachoen* [...] *Gal. lat.* 1490 *alchohen* (cap. 26, *de alchohen*).

(3) *Alfagdi* [...] *Rasis* [...] *exponit quod agnus castus idem est in libro G. de simplici medicina liber .vi. capitulo de agno casto. Alfagdi* [...] Rhazes [...] explains that it is agnus castus, and it is the same in Galen's book on *Simple Medicines*, book six, chapter on agnus castus.

In this case the Latin translation has a different term (glossed by agnus castus) in cap. 2 (*de agno casto*), but I am too uncertain of the spelling to provide a transliteration here.

(4) *Alguasen* [...]. *Et etiam G. i.vi. de simplici medicina, ubi dicit quod sic vocatur propter iuvamentum quod efficit in morsu canis rabiosi* [...]*Alguasen* [...]. And also Galen, in the sixth book of *Simple medicines* where he says that it is called thus in the context of it treating the bite of a rabid dog [...]
(Gal. *alusson* K. XI, 823)
Gal. lat. 1490 *alusen*, under cap. 24 *de alusen*.
Pal. lat. 1094 f. 554v *alusen*
Cf. Ullmann, p. 96 (same term for Al-Bitriq and Hunain, translit. from the Greek)

(5) *Anchusa* [...] *Alia ancusa quam multi albucidion vocant supradicta parvior est* [...] *G. in .vi. de simplici medicina quattuor eius ponit species, una vocatur ibi simar, alia locasus, tertia abugelabus quartam dicit carere nomine, et omnia ista nomina sunt greco corrupta* [...][25]*Anchusa* [...]. Another *ancusa*, which is often called *albucidion*, is smaller than the one mentioned above [...] Galen mentions four species of it in the sixth book of *Simple Medicines*, one is called *simiar* there, the other *locasus*, the third *abugelabus*. He says that the fourth does not have a name, and all these names are corrupt in the Greek [...]
Gal. lat. 1490 vol. 2 (119) has all the words cited here under cap. 4 *de lactuca asini*.
Pal. lat. 1094 f. 552v (same except for *locassus*, instead of *locasus*).
See below n. 9 (*lactuca asini*) and section 3 with the Greek text on *anchusa*.

(6) *Almalke in .vi. G. de simplicibus medicinis est* [...]Almalke is in the sixth book of Galen's *Simple medicines* [...]
Gal. lat. 1490 vol. 2: *almalhe*, cap. 22 *de almalhe*

---

25 *Simar* AC | *syniar* B | *stimar* e | *simax* f.

(7) *Canicalnemer in .vi. Ga. de simplicibus medicis, est inquit strangulator leopardi et cetera, est species achoniti. Canicalnemer* is mentioned in the sixth book of Galen's *Simple medicines*, and he says: 'it is *strangulator leopardi*' and so on, it is a species of *achonitum*.
Gal. lat. 1490 vol. 2 (120) cap. 19 *de strangulatore leopardi sive achonito. Canichalnemer* or *Chainchalnemer*
Missing in *Pal. lat.* 1094
Wrong transcription from the Arabic, see Ullmann p. 501.

(8) *Sibar in .vi. Gal. in simplicibus medicinis scribitur pro sarb quod est aloes. Sibar* is written in the sixth book of Galen's Simple Medicines for *sarb*, which is *aloes*.
Gal. *Simple medicines* XI, 821 *aloes*
Gal. lat. 1490 vol. 2 (120) cap. 23 *de aloe. Sybar.*
Pal. lat. 1094 (s. XIV) f. 554r *Cibar.*
Cf. Ullmann p. 95

(9) *Lactuca asini* [...] *Gal. vero in sexto de simplicibus medicinis .iiii. dicit esse eius species, quarum unam vocat onocalia, secundam locasus, tertiam abugelabus quartam dicit carere nomine et omnes dicit esse species asinar, de his supra in abugilisse.*[26] *Lactuca asini* [...] but Galen in the sixth book of *Simple Medicines* says that there are four species, one of which he calls *onocalia*, the second *locasus*, the third *abugelabus*. He says the fourth does not have a name, and he says that all are a type of *asinar*, on these see above under *abugilisse*.
Gal. lat. 1490 vol. 2 (119) has all the words cited here unde cap. 4 *de lactuca asini*
Pal. lat. 1094 f. 552v (same except for *locassus*).
Cf. Ullmann p. 72

(10) *Melha* [...] *Galie. in libro de simplici medicina in sexto vocat almalhe. Melha* [...] in the sixth book of *Simple Medicines* calls it *alhalhe*."
Gal. *Simple medicines* XI, 821 *alimon*
Gal. lat. 1490 vol. 2 (120) has *almalhe* under cap. 22 *de almalhe*
Pal. lat. 1094 f. 554r *almalhe*
Cf. Ullmann p. 94 (Hunain vs. Al-Bitriq)

(11) *Suchaha* [...] *G. vero in sexto de simplici medicina dicit suchaha habere virtutem bedorad* [...] *Suchaha* [...] but Galen in the sixth book on *Simple Medicines* says that *suchaha* has the same properties as *bedorad* [...]
Gal. *Simple med.* XI, 819 *akanthos aiguptias*

---

26 *Asinar* AC | *asiniar* B e | i *add. supra lineam* f.

Gal. lat. 1490 vol. 2 (120) cap. 17 *de spina Arabica. Ancaha. Bedeoard.*
Pal. lat. 1094 f. 553v *sucdaha?*
Cf. Ullmann p. 85 (orthographic variation in Arabic)

(12) *Sentix est rubus Gal. li. de simplici medicina radicem eius inter medicinas frangentes lapidem enumerat et est rubus .s. batus. Sentix* is blackberry, Galen in *Simple Medicines* lists its root amongst the medicines that break up stones, and it is blackberry, that is *batus.*
Gal. 1490 ch. 75 *de rubo bato.*

(13) *Semabras* [...] *exponitur a Gal. in .vi. de simplici medicina circa primum quod est salamandra* [...] *Semabras* [...] it is described by Galen in the sixth book of *Simple Medicines* around the beginning that it is *salamandra.*
Galen provides no definition of *salamandra* in his treatise *Simple medicines.*
(14) *Iantum vel ientum ut in .iiii. Gal. de simplici medicina, ubi numerat quedam que non licet gustare est psia ut apparet per Sera. ca. de tapsia et infra vocant ipsum gingizerd.*[27] *Iantum* or *Ientum* as in the fourth book of Galen's *Simple Medicines,* where he lists things one should not taste, says it is *psia,* as it appears from Serapion, chapter on *tapsia,* and below they call it *gingizerd.*

The origin of the Latin translation is unclear. Richard Durling, who has studied in depth the Latin Galen, changed his mind over time about the translation of Galen's *Simple medicines.* He ascribed first the translation to Constantinus Africanus, then to Gerard of Cremona. The evidence for such an attribution is, in fact, thin: one of the manuscripts (*Pal. lat.* 1092, f. 22ra) ascribes the translation to Gerard. But this mention belongs to the first part of the text, and we cannot be certain that the same authorship applies to the second part, Books VI-XI.[28] An in-depth study of this Latin translation from book one to eleven would certainly be illuminating. However remote this prospect may be, even a preliminary study of this translation yields interesting results. First of all, the translation of Book VI (unlike other books) specifies one thing: the name of the author of the Arabic translation, Hunain son of Isaac, thus supporting the common opinion, also apparent in Arabic manuscripts, that Hunain translated *Simple medicines,* not his

27 *Iantum* vel *ientum* AC | *Iantam* vel *gentum* vel *alientum* B | *Iantum* vel *gentum* vel *aligentum* e | *Iantum* vel *ientum* vel *alientum* f. *Et infra vocant ipsum gingizerd* AC | om. B ef.
28 Two manuscripts (*Pal. lat.* 1092, f. 22ra; Krakow 800, information courtesy of Stefania Fortuna) ascribe the translation to Gerard.

nephew Hubaish – but that is a debated question.[29] Secondly, the translation reflects a different bipartition than I expected.

As it happens, the material gathered by Durling (kindly put at my disposal by Stefania Fortuna) shows that a wealth of manuscripts have the Arabo-Latin translation of Books I-V, but very few contain Book VI and none have a full translation from the Arabic. In fact, Durling mentions manuscripts transmitting Books I-VI, or parts of Book VI alone, but no additional books. It is one of those few manuscripts (the *Pal. lat.* 1094) that I consulted next to the printed edition of 1490 to gain an insight of this translation.[30] This manuscript is usually dated from the fourteenth century and has a lot of marginal annotations (unfortunately, they are illegible on the poor printouts from microfilm which I have at my disposal). The other three manuscripts mentioned by Durling are of a similar date; they are Kues *Hospital* 297 (s. XIII-XIV), *Par. lat.* 9331 (s. XIV), and *Vat. lat.* 2385 (s. ?). I consulted the *Par. lat.* 9331 on microfilm.[31]

In fact, the translation of Books VII-XI published by Bonardus in 1490 is based on a Greek rather than an Arabic source. It is thus clear that Bonardus followed two different sources: one for Books I-VI (an Arabo-Latin translation), one for Books VII-XI (a Greco-Latin translation). He may have simply brought together two different translations: one made after a model in Arabic (Books I-VI), one made after a Greek one (VII-XI), probably later. He may also have used a Latin manuscript in which such a combination was made, as in the *Par. lat.* 9331.[32] The second section (Books VII-XI) is perhaps a part of the translation of Books VI-XI ascribed to Niccolo da Reggio. At any rate, Simon cannot have used the Greco-Latin translation, which was probably made decades after his death.[33] But it is a fact that some manuscripts contain only Book VI of Galen's *Simple medicines* in the Arabo-Latin translation ascribed to Gerardus of Cremona. It is therefore no wonder that Simon of Genoa should quote and even mention only Book VI

---

29 Cf. Ullmann, Wörterbuch..., Ivan Garofalo, "Un sondaggio sul *De simplicium medicamentorum facultate* di Galeno." in Clelia Sarnelli Cerqua (Ed.) *Studi arabo-islamici in onore di Roberto Rubinacci nel suo settantesimo compleanno*, (Napoli: Istituto Universitario Orientale, 1985), 317-325.

30 Galeni opera, Flippo Pinzi, 1490. The edition was curated by Diomedes Bonardus.

31 I owe additional information on these manuscripts and others to Stefania Fortuna, who is preparing the online catalogue of the Latin Galen; see my forthcoming article mentioned note 16. My inspection of a microfilm of Kues *Hospital* 297 shows that the manuscript contains books I-V of Gerardus' translation only.

32 According to my provisional observations, Bonardus could have used the *Par lat.* 9331, which displays exactly the same pattern; but some differences between the manuscript and the edition show that it wasn't his only source.

33 I. Ventura gives evidence to date the translation of Galen's Simples before 1332, based on Matteo Silvatico's *Liber pandectarum*; see Ventura Iolanda, Cultura medica a Napoli nel XIV secolo. In: *Boccaccio Angioino*. (Bruxelles, Lang, 2012), 251-288 (esp. p. 286).

of Galen's *Simple medicines*: it is possible that he accessed only Book VI in the Latin manuscripts at his disposal. It looks as if only Books I-VI were available in the thirteenth century; it is even possible that the translation of Book VI was available in separate manuscripts, as an excerpt; moreover, it may have been made separately from the other first five books. There is a notable difference in the Latin translation between Book VI and the other five books: it is only at the beginning of Book VI that Hunain is named as a translator; no such mention appears in the earlier books. Only a detailed stylistic study will help decide whether we deal with a distinct translation for Book VI. At any rate, the fact that Book VI circulated separately could explain why Simon seems unaware of the rest of the text.

The last two examples above (thirteen and fourteen), however, pose me a problem: I could not identify a mention of *salamandra* in Book VI in Greek; and I don't understand the topic of the last example, which refers to either Book IV, or Chapter IV in Book VI (cf. ex. 9). Of course, it would be helpful to be able to decide whether Simon actually also read Book IV. But overall, our evidence points to Book VI as the sole source used by Simon.

Looking at the evidence from the textual transmission of *Simple medicines*, it is clear that Simon used an older, but similar source to the Latin edition and manuscript I was able to check. Little variation is found between the 'quotations' in the *Clavis* and the Latin translation of *Simple medicines* Book VI as we know it, apart from slight variations in the spelling. This variation may be due to textual transmission problems, or to unstable methods in transliterating Arabic words. The Arabic terms studied by Ullmann in two different Arabic translations of Book VI, one by Al-Bitriq and one by Hunain, show that there can be slight spelling differences for the same word even in Arabic. Also, a comparison between the terms appearing in the Latin translation and the two Arabic versions shows that the Latin translator used the translation ascribed to Hunain and not Al-Bitriq (who relies more heavily on transliterations from the Greek). The latter probably never reached the West.

Simon's occasional quotations of Galen's *Simple medicines* do not contribute to our knowledge of its transmission. Indeed, we have several Arabic manuscripts and a few reliable Greek ones of roughly the same period as Simon: the Latin translation and Simon's quotations thus look like secondary material. As for Galen's place in Simon's project: it seems to be quite limited. There are less than fifteen explicit mentions of *Simple Medicines* Book VI in the *Clavis*. As is clear from the examples provided, Galen's text is usually abruptly summarized and used along other sources that feature more prominently in the *Clavis*, such as Pliny, Avicenna, Serapion, or Dioscorides. Simon actually states clearly in his preface that he disagrees with Galen about the importance of plant names (for all his philological sense, Galen did not want to put nomenclature forward in his treatise on simples). As I have shown in this brief study, however, the poor availability of Galen's text at the time explains in great part Simon's apparent lack of interest in his terminology and method. The theoretical part (Books I-V) of Galen's treatise may never have reached him in any language, and Books VII-XI certainly didn't.

It is important to realize that the Latin translation made from the Arabic was at times fairly remote from the original Greek text; there could be a number of reasons for this, such as the manifold stages of translation (from Greek to Syriac, then Arabic, then Latin), or the problems of transliteration and copying. At any rate, the relative rarity of many a plant name in Galen's catalogue certainly proved an aggravating factor. In order to illustrate what must have been an additional difficulty for Simon's enterprise, I would like to compare more closely a Greek passage from Book VI with Simon's reading of the Latin translation. I have selected Chapter VI, 4 about a kind of bugloss, a plant from the family of the *Boraginaceae* of which the various species have entailed confusion even in modern nomenclature.[34] This brief case study shows that such confusion was already strong in ancient texts.

I append (see annexe) a small sample edition of the Greek (namely Chapter 4 of Book VI, on *anchusa*). Naturally, this is all provisional, based on the essential manuscripts at our disposal. It is tempting to contrast the Greek chapter with Simon's Lemmas 5 and 9 (above) about *anchusa* and *lactuca asini* or *asinar*. In Lemma 5, Simon points out the four species of *anchusa* mentioned by Galen together with their names, but ends up saying that all those names are 'corrupt in Greek' (*greco corrupta*). Where the Greek has ὀνόκλεια, λυκαψὸς, ὀνόχειλος, and Ἀλκιβιαδεῖον, in Latin Simon mentions (Lemma 5) *simar*, *locasus*, *abugelabus*, and one anonymous species (but he also adds the name of *albucidion*); in another lemma (9), he provides in addition *onocalia* next to *locasus* and *abugelabus* as species of *asinar*. Indeed, the terms *simar*, *locasus*, and *abugelabus* (and even *onocalia*, albeit closer to the Greek) transferred from Arabic and did not necessarily ring a bell for someone familiar with Greek pharmacopeia, Simon prefers to use Avicenna's terms, which he deemed more reliable, probably because they had grown more common and were widely used; unlike the terms used in Galen's Book VI as transmitted in a Latin version. When you read this chapter in Greek in the Kühn edition, you may indeed believe at first sight, like Simon, that the names are corrupt: twice in the same chapter, one can read λύκοψις, instead of the original form λυκαψὸς. But in this case, as the apparatus shows, the Greek manuscripts provide all the necessary material to edit the text correctly; neither the Arabic, nor the Latin are of any help. At any

34 *Cf.* Selvi, Federico, Nardi, Enio and Massimo Bigazzi, "The ultimate types of *Anchusa L.* and *Lycopsis L.* (Boraginaceae)." *Taxon* 45 (1996): 305-307.

rate, the Arabo-Latin translation gives a poor rendering of the Greek terms; it is no wonder that Simon should have found the plant names 'corrupt'. For Simon, the Latin translation obscured the original text more than it revealed it; and even Avicenna got the Greek *alkibiadeion* wrong, if we are to trust the mixed-up form *albucidon* cited by Simon in the same passage. The various species of *anchusa* (and their names) are an example of poor transmission via the medieval Arabic and Latin translations. The correct names of the four *anchusai* actually appear in Dioscorides, not just in Galen, but this fact, too, escaped Simon's research. One century later, he could have read a more complete text. But even then, the Latin translation of Galen's treatise *Simple Medicines* in its entirety could barely be completed, and it certainly failed to become widely available.[35] Contrary to what I would have expected then, Galen's treatise *Simple medicines*, which had become a classic in the Islamic world, may have reached a similar status in the medieval West only later.

---

[35] Virtually all medieval Latin manuscripts have only a partial text, unless the treatise was artificially completed by using two different translations (Books I-V or I-VI from the Arabic, the remaining books from the Greek). An exception lies in ms. *Urbinas lat.* 248, which, according to R. Durling (information courtesy of Stefania Fortuna), has preserved a complete Latin translation from the Greek: six manuscripts provide a combination of both the Arabo-Latin and the Greco-Latin translations: they are *Par. lat.* 9331, Paris, *Académie de médecine 52 and 53*, *Vat. lat.* 2388, Dresden, *SLUB* Db 92-93, Erfurt, *Universitätsbibliothek* 278. On the importance of this translation, ascribed to Niccolò da Reggio: see my forthcoming study (mentioned note 16) of the Latin tradition of Galen's *Simple medicines.*

Bibliography

Cavallo, Guglielmo. "La trasmissione scritta della cultura greca antica in Calabria e in Sicilia tra i secoli X e XV: Consistenza, tipologia, fruizione." *Scrittura e Civiltà* 4 (1980): 157-245.

Claudii Galeni Opera Omnia (1821-1833), edited by C.G. Kühn.

Dickson, Keith. *Stephanus the philosopher and physician: commentary on Galen's* Therapeutics to Glaucon. *Introd., Greek text with critical apparatus and index of sources, English transl., notes.* Leiden: Brill, 1998.

Everett, Nicholas. *The Alphabet of Galen. Pharmacy from Antiquity to the Middle Ages.* Toronto: University of Toronto Press, 2011.

Fichtner, Gerhard. *Corpus Galenicum. Ein Verzeichnis der galenischen und pseudo-galenischen Schriften.* Tübingen, 2011, accessible online on the website of the *Corpus Medicorum Graecorum* in Berlin http://cmg.bbaw.de/online-publications/Galen-Bibliographie_2012_08_28.pdf

Garofalo, Ivan. "Un sondaggio sul *De simplicium medicamentorum facultate* di Galeno." In Clelia Sarnelli Cerqua (Ed.) *Studi arabo-islamici in onore di Roberto Rubinacci nel suo settantesimo compleanno.* Napoli: Istituto Universitario Orientale, 1985, 317-325.

— "La traduzione araba dei compendi alessandrini delle opere del canone di Galeno. Il compendio dell'Ad Glauconem." *Medicina nei Secoli N.S.* 6 (1994): 329–348.

Ieraci Bio, Anna Maria. "La trasmissione della letteratura medica greca nell'Italia meridionale fra X e XV secolo." In Antonio Garzya (Ed.), *Contributi alla cultura Greca nell'Italia meridionale.* Naples: Bibliopolis, 1989, 133-255.

Irigoin, Jean. "La tradition de l'*Ars medica* de Galien dans l'Italie méridionale." *Bollettino della Badia graeca di Grottaferrata* N.S. 45 (1991): 85-91.

Löfstedt, Bengt. "Zum Lateinischen Kommentar von Galens Ad Glauconem." In Jozsef Herman (Ed.), *Latin vulgaire – latin tardif. Actes du Ier Colloque international sur le latin vulgaire et tardif (Pécs, 2–5 septembre 1985)*. Tübingen: Niemeyer, 1987, 145–151.

Nutton, Vivian. "Medicine in Late Antiquity and the Early Middle Ages." In Lawrence I. Conrad et al. (Eds.), *The Western Medical Tradition*. Cambridge: Cambridge University Press, 1995, reprint 2007, 71-87.

Opsomer-Halleux, Carmelia. "Un herbier médicinal du haut moyen-âge: l'*alfabetum galieni*." *History and Philosophy of the Life Sciences* 4 (1982): 65-97.

Petit, Caroline. "Théorie et pratique: connaissance et diffusion du traité des *Simples* de Galien au Moyen Age." In Arsenio Ferraces Rodríguez (Ed.), *Fitozooterapia antigua y altomedieval : textos y doctrinas*. A Coruña: Univ. da Coruña, Servizo de Publicacións, 2009, 79-95.

— "La tradition manuscrite du traité des Simples de Galien. *Editio princeps* et traduction annotée des chapitres 1 à 3 du livre I." In Véronique Boudon-Millot, Jouanna Jouanna, Antonio Garzya and Amneris Roselli (Eds.), *Histoire de la tradition et édition des médecins grecs - Storia della tradizione e edizione dei medici greci*. Napoli: D'Auria, 2010, 143-165.

Selvi, Federico, Enio Nardi and Massimo Bigazzi. "The ultimate types of *Anchusa L.* and *Lycopsis L.* (Boraginaceae)." *Taxon* 45 (1996): 305-307.

Ullmann, Manfred. *Wörterbuch zu den griechisch-arabischen Übersetzungen des neunten Jahrhunderts*. Wiesbaden: Harrassowitz, 2002.

Appendix:

A case study: Gal. *Simple med.* VI, 4 (XI, 811-813 K.). Working edition.

<u>Sigla</u>:
Vatican, *BAV Urbinas* gr. 67 =U, s. XIII (f. 192v-193r)
Vatican, *BAV Pal.* gr. 31 = Pal, s. XIV (?) (f. 80 rv)
Vatican, *BAV Barberinus* I, 127 = Barb, s. XV (f. 209rv)
N.B.: readings here ascribed to Kühn sometimes date back to earlier printed
editions, such as Chartier's 1639 edition (vol. XIII).

VI. 4. 1.δ΄. Περὶ ἀγχούσης [καὶ τεττάρων ἀγχουσῶν]. 2. Τῆς δὲ ἀγχούσης
τέτταρά ἐστιν εἴδη, ὧν ἡ μὲν ὀνομαζομένη **ὀνόκλεια** ψύχουσαν ἱκανῶς καὶ
ξηραίνουσαν ἔχει τὴν ῥίζαν, στύφουσάν τε ἅμα καὶ ὑπόπικρον, ἱκανὴν δὲ [καὶ]
λεπτῦναι καὶ ἀπορρῦψαι τοὺς χολώδεις χυμοὺς καὶ πυκνῶσαι τὰ σώματα.
τὰ δὲ φύλλα ἀσθενέστερα μὲν ἔχει τῆς ῥίζης, στύφει δὲ αὐτὰ καὶ ξηραίνει.
3. καὶ ἡ **λυκαψὸς** δὲ προσαγορευομένη ψύχει μὲν καὶ ξηραίνει, ῥίζαν δ᾽
ἔχει στυπτικωτέραν τῆς ὀνοκλείας. 4. ἡ δὲ **ὀνόχειλος** θερμοτέρα τέ ἐστι
καὶ φαρμακωδεστέρα. Πλέον γὰρ ἔχει καὶ πρὸς τὴν γεῦσιν εὐθὺς τὸ δριμύ.
ταύτης δ᾽ ἔτι θερμοτέρα, ἡ τετάρτη καὶ μικρὰ καὶ πικροτέρα καὶ πλέον ἔτι
φαρμακωδεστέρα τυγχάνει. 5. ἄγχουσαι δὲ οὐ τῆς αὐτῆς ἅπασαι δυνάμεως.
ἡ μὲν γὰρ **ὀνόκλεια** προσαγορευομένη στύφουσάν τε ἅμα καὶ ὑπόπικρον
ἔχει τὴν ῥίζαν, ἱκανὴν καὶ πυκνῶσαι τὰ σώματα καὶ μετρίως λεπτῦναι καὶ
ἀπορρῦψαι καὶ ἀποπλῦναι τοὺς χολώδεις καὶ ἀλμυρώδεις χυμούς. 6. ἐρρέθη
γὰρ ἐν τοῖς ἔμπροσθεν ὡς ἡ στρυφνὴ ποιότης ἐπιμεμιγμένη τῇ πικρᾷ ταῦτα
ἐργάζεσθαι πέφυκεν. οὕτω τέ τοι καὶ ἰκτερικοῖς καὶ σπληνικοῖς καὶ νεφριτικοῖς
ὠφέλιμος ὑπάρχει. ἔστι δὲ καὶ ψύχειν μὲν ἱκανὴ καὶ καταπλασσομένη γε σὺν
ἀλφίτοις ἐρυσιπέλασι ὠφελεῖ, καὶ ἀπορρύπτει δὲ οὐ πινομένη μόνον, ἀλλὰ
κα⟨ὶ⟩ ἔξωθεν ἐπιτιθεμένη, καὶ διὰ τοῦτο καὶ ἀλφοὺς καὶ λέπρας ἰᾶται σὺν ὄξει.
7. τὰ μὲν τῆς ῥίζης ἔργα ταῦτα καὶ αἱ τῶν ἔργων δυνάμεις αἱ εἰρημέναι. τὰ
δὲ φύλλα τῆς βοτάνης ἐστὶν μὲν ἀσθενέστερα τῆς ῥίζης, οὐκ ἀπήλλακται δὲ
τοῦ ξηραίνειν τε καὶ στύφειν, ὥστε καὶ διάρροιας ἰᾶται σὺν οἴνω πινόμενα.
8. ⟨καὶ ἡ **λυκαψὸς** δὲ προσαγορευομένη τοῖς ἐρυσιπέλασιν ὁμοίως ἁρμόττει
καὶ ῥίζαν ἔχει στυπτικωτέραν τῆς ὀνοκλείας. 9. τῆς δὲ **ὀνοχείλου** τε καὶ
Ἀλκιβιαδείου καλουμένης ἡ μὲν δύναμίς ἐστι φαρμακωδεστέρα. πλέον γοῦν
ἔχει καὶ πρὸς τὴν γεῦσιν εὐθὺς τὸ δριμὺ καὶ ἐχεοδήκτοις ἱκανῶς ἁρμόττει
καταπλαττομένη καὶ περιαπτομένη καὶ ἐσθιομένη. 10. λοιπὴ δὲ ἡ τετάρτη
καὶ μικρὰ καὶ σχεδὸν ἀνώνυμος ἐξ αὐτῶν μόνη, παραπλησία μέν ἐστι τῇ
Ἀλκιβιαδείω, πικροτέρα δὲ καὶ πλέον ἐστὶ φαρμακωδεστέρα, καὶ διὰ τοῦτο
πρὸς τὰς πλατείας ἕλμινθας ἐπιτηδεία, πλῆθος ὀξυβάφου σὺν ὑσσώπω τε καὶ
καρδάμω πινομένη.

VI. 4. 1-4 def. in Pal

VI. 4. 1. post ἀγχούσης add. καὶ τεττάρων ἀγχουσῶν Kühn || Περὶ ἀγχούσης om. Pal || 2. τέτταρά ἐστιν εἴδη U: τέτταρά εἰσιν εἴδη Barb τέταρτόν ἐστιν εἶδος Kühn|| ὀνομαζομένη om. U Kühn|| ἱκανῶς om. U|| ἱκανὴν Barb Kühn: -ὸν U|| καὶ add. Kühn|| 3. λυκαψὸς Barb: λυκαῖος (?) U λύκοψις Kühn|| στυπτικωτέραν τῆς ὀνοκλείας U Kühn: τῆς ὀνοκλείας στυπτικωτέραν Barb || 4. πλέον γὰρ ἔχει καὶ πρὸς τὴν γεῦσιν εὐθὺς τὸ δριμύ Barb Kühn: πρὸς τὴν γεῦσιν δὲ πλέον ἔχει εὐθὺς τὸ δριμύ U|| ἡ τετάρτη om. Kühn|| καὶ U Barb: ἢ Kühn|| ἔτι om. U|| ἄγχουσαι δὲ οὐ τῆς αὐτῆς ἄπασαι δυνάμεως Pal Kühn: ἄγχουσαι τέσσαρες οὐ τῆς αὐτῆς ἄπασαι δυνάμεως Barb οὐ τῆς αὐτῆς δ' ἄπασαι δυνάμεως U|| τε om. U|| ἁλμυρώδεις Pal Kühn: ἁλμώδεις Barb ἁλμύδεις U|| 6. ἐπιμεμιγμένη Pal Kühn ἐπιμιγνυμένη U Barb || τέ om. Barb || νεφριτικοῖς Pal U Kühn: νεφρικοῖς Barb || μὲν om. U|| γε Pal Kühn: τε U γέ τοι Barb || ἐρυσιπέλασι U Barb: ἐρυσιπέλατ Pal ἐρυσιπέλατα Kühn|| 7. τὰ μὲν τῆς ῥίζης ἔργα U Pal Kühn: τὰ μὲν τῆς αὐτῆς ἔργα ῥίζης Barb || αἱ om. U|| τῆς βοτάνης om. U|| τε om. U|| διάρροιας U Barb: -αν Pal Kühn || σὺν οἴνῳ πινόμενα U Pal Kühn: πινόμενον σὺν οἴνῳ Barb || 8. λυκαψὸς Pal Barb: λύκαψος U λύκοψις Kühn || ἁρμόττει U Barb ἁρμόζει Pal Kühn || 9. ὀνοχείλου U Pal: - ος Barb -ους Kühn || τε om. U|| Ἀλκιβιαδείου Kühn: -αδίου Pal -άδος U Barb || γοῦν Pal Kühn: οὖν U Barb || ἐχεοδήκτοις codd.: ἔχι. Kühn || περιαπτομένη καὶ ἐσθιομένη Pal Kühn: ἐσθιομένη καὶ περιαπτομένη U Barb || 10. λοιπὴ δὲ ἡ codd.: ἡ λοιπὴ δὲ Kühn || Ἀλκιβιαδείῳ Kühn: -δίῳ Pal -άδι U Barb || ἐστὶ Pal Kühn: ἔτι Barb om. U.

Barbara Zipser

Simon Online, an Alternative Approach to Research and Publishing

The idea to create *Simon Online* was born many years ago when I was a doctoral student at the University of Heidelberg. Having obtained a photocopy of the *Clavis sanationis*, a vast Latin-Greek-Arabic medical dictionary from the late thirteenth-century papal court, it quickly became clear that this was an extremely important work and needed to be looked at in more detail, and that it would not be possible to do so in any of the conventional scenarios.

Such a project would require a wide and flexible collaboration between highly specialized scholars, and in addition, would run over a long period of time. Moreover, it would be necessary to establish patterns in the text before embarking on an edition; we would need to search the material in a very efficient way, for instance to identify spelling conventions or the way primary sources were selected.

Some years later, a project draft for *Simon Online* was accepted as part of a Wellcome Trust University Award.[1] The idea was to make raw material – in this case a transcription and photographs of primary sources – available online, and open the project up for scholars to edit the text and add commentaries and translations to entries they are particularly interested in.

The first, very easy step, was to set up the database and upload a transcription of the text based on an early modern printing, which had been completed by Thomas Smith. I then added templates, an index, and help pages, wrote a few sample entries and announced the project. After a few weeks, others joined in and more and more entries appeared. Currently, 839 entries have been edited.[2]

These entries are then being copy-edited to even out the formatting. In a final step, keywords in these entries are added to various indices; the most important of these is the index rerum,[3] which list the topics discussed. These are two snippets from the index to the letter *A*:

---

1 Grant number 048921.

2 A list of these entries can be found here: http://www.simonofgenoa.org/index.php5?title=Translated_entries

3 http://www.simonofgenoa.org/index.php5?title=Index_rerum

'Aconitum, Acorn, Active, Agnus castus...'

'Anise, Ant, Antelope, Antichrist,[4] Aphrodisiac, Apple, Aquamarine, Arsenic, Artemisia...'

Most of the entries in the *Clavis* cover medicinal plants. Some describe diseases, surgical instruments (for instance transurethral catheters), or other medical terminology.

Simon Online also provides other indices, for instance a list of scientific plant names, place names, and authors quoted. The latter category can also be used to reconstruct sources, e.g. a mysterious *Liber de doctrina graeca* or *Book on Greek study* that cannot be identified with any known text and that has been all but forgotten by academia.

Perhaps more unusual are the index categories 'Interviews' and 'Known Unknowns'; these pages list entries, in which Simon asks native speakers for advice if he is unsure about the meaning of a word, and in which he states that the evidence is inconclusive. These entries are invaluable for both linguists – as they give us a first hand account of the pronunciation of a given word – and medical historians and pharmacologists – as they allow us to identify medicinal plants used at the time.

His interviewees are no less of interest. Simon consulted, for instance, at least two native speakers of Arabic, whom he describes as 'an Arabic woman from Aleppo,[5] who had sufficient experience with herbs' and 'another woman from a different region'.[6] Unfortunately, he does not tell us where he met these women, but his account still gives a glimpse of the world in which Simon lived and worked. Arabic was not a dead language to

---

4 This word appears in the entry *D littera*, Simon's explanation of how the letter 'd' could be pronounced in various languages. Of all Greek words starting with *anti-* he chose 'antichrist' to illustrate that 't' could under certain circumstances sound like 'd'.

5 This woman is described in two entries, **Achavě** and *Handacocha*, as [...] *saracena de alef* [...]' a Saracen woman from Alef'. The town name is also transmitted as Haleph in B in the entry **Achavě**. Both Siam Bhayro and Werner Arnold confirm that this could indeed be Aleppo, and I am very grateful for their professional expertize in the matter. Arnold also suggests that the name could refer to Tell Halaf near Edessa. The town name Alef or Haleph is as such not attested, but it could according to Bhayro be explained via a Hebrew intermediary, or according to Arnold via a Syriac form. Syriac was at this point still widely spoken in rural areas. According to Arnold, the dialect of the woman from Alef is consistent with the urban dialect of Aleppo. I obtained a copy of Yann Dahhaoui *L'atelier de Simon de Genes. Vers une edition de la Clavis sanationis.* (MA thesis, Lausanne, 2001), after this article had been submitted. On p. 128, he also discusses the Arabic women, and identifies the town name as Aleppo.

6 She is mentioned in the entry **Achavě**. Intriguingly, when asked how a specific plant is called, she gave three synonyms, one of which would according to Werner Arnold would be consistent with the rural dialect of Syria.

him, and he did not solely rely on books.[7] He was also approachable and communicative.[8]

These are just two gems one finds when digging deep enough in the database. Simon also describes other curious findings: he saw papyrus scrolls held by monastery libraries in Rome, which appear to be written in cursive handwriting.[9] He is also the only person to have described a sole surviving manuscript of a Herophilean text on eye diseases.[10]

*

From the start, the main aim of the project was to provide a resource for Classicists who may not read Arabic (and vice versa), and to make the material accessible to scientists who may not be fluent in Latin, the main language of the *Clavis*. This last group may in fact have an interest in this type of material, even though its content may appear outdated at first sight: traditional herbal medications can be screened for active ingredients.

However, the process of identifying a plant can be very complicated indeed in Medieval texts. At the time the *Clavis* was composed, the medical literature available could be written in at least three languages: Latin, Greek, and Arabic. Of these writings, the Latin and Greek evidence could have been composed several centuries ago. Moreover, Latin texts did not necessarily have their origins in a romance language country, as it was widely used as a language of scholarly discourse. And even if a Latin text was in fact written in Italy, the vegetation may have changed since the composition of the text, which could in turn lead to wrong conclusions. To complicate matters, many Medieval Latin sources

---

7 Simon was indeed able to understand Arabic, as is clear from the entry *Corrat Alhayn*, where he overhears Arabic speakers making compliments to women. He seems to have had, however, only limited reading skills when it came to Arabic script. For instance, in the entry *Usnen* he seems to believe that the Arabic *alif* was always pronounced as 'a' (see also *Asnen*). Simon was also able to converse with members of other linguistic groups. In the entry *Mahaleb*, he talks to Spanish people (who speak Spanish, rather than Arabic).

8 See for instance the entry *Iris*, where an Arabic soldier asks him for help in identifying a presumably Latin word called *irse*. Simon identifies it correctly as a misspelled *iris* when he sees it in Arabic letters.

9 See *Kirtas*: [...] *et ego vidi Rome in gazofilatiis antiquorum monasteriorum libros et privilegia ex hac materia scripta ex litteris apud nos non intelligibilibus, nam figure nec ex toto grece nec ex toto latine erant.* '[...] and I saw in Rome in the treasure chambers of the old monasteries books and documents that were made of this material (sc. papyrus) with letters that are not intelligible to us, for the characters were neither entirely Greek nor entirely Latin.' The script Simon is referring to could be found in both books and *privilegia*, most likely papal documents.

10 For an in depth analysis see: Heinrich von Staden, *Herophilus. The Art of Medicine in Early Alexandria*. (Cambridge: Cambridge University Press, 1989), 570 ff.

are translations of Greek or Arabic texts, or a Latin translation of an Arabic intermediary of a lost Greek source. Evidently, such scenarios involved many different geographical areas, and are bound to lead to misunderstandings.

Such a situation can also arise in the descriptions of very common medicinal herbs, for instance *pulegium*, which is commonly identified as pennyroyal. This plant is mentioned in twenty-nine entries of the *Clavis*, discussing its name in various languages, and other plants it could potentially be confused with. This last point was crucial, as it could, according to the sources, look like certain types of basil or mint. Pennyroyal had become somewhat of a running gag in Classical Greek comedy as it was amongst others used to induce abortions, and it is frequently mentioned in medicinal texts.[11]

The uncertainty about the external appearance of these plants probably has its roots in the rate of mutation, as Wilf Gunther, one of the authors on *Simon Online*, writes in the entry on *mentastrum*, a plant that was also called 'wild *pulegium*': '...The ability of most mints to escape from cultivation and to hybridise makes the botanical identification of *mentastrum* difficult.'

In addition, the written tradition, and in particular the translation to and from the Arabic had managed to cause considerable confusion, and having discussed the evidence extensively, Simon decided to double-check. In the entry *Gliconium* he writes: '...Similarly it says in the old *Book on simple medicines* that the Greeks call pennyroyal *gliconos*. I asked a Greek person, and he says it was called *vliconos*, and this is also what it says in the *Book on Greek study*.' He later continues: 'Little wonder the Arabs make mistakes with these plants that have a similar appearance and power.'[12]

---

11 For an overview, see John M. Riddle, "Oral Contraceptives and Early-Term Abortifacients during Classical Antiquity and the Middle Ages." *Past and Present* 132 (August 1991): 18-32.

12 *Vliconos* is, in any spelling, not attested. The *Clavis* also contains several more Greek words that are not attested in other sources. Perhaps the most striking are *Vatrachi kampite* (entry edited by Dionysios Stathakopoulos) and *Miosos* (edited by Barbara Zipser), both types of frogs. If these entries reflect vocabulary Simon overheard in everyday life, then he must have seen the frogs in question, as both entries are very detailed. Alternatively, they could be quoted from a dictionary. This is less likely for two reasons: firstly, Simon usually adds a reference to his quotes. Second, his word for 'field-frog' is clearly a medieval vernacular term. This idiom was very rarely used in writing, and to my knowledge there are no zoological books or dictionaries extant from this time. The word is not attested in Ioannes archiatrus, as edited in Barbara Zipser, *John the Physician's Therapeutics: A Medical Handbook in Vernacular Greek*. (Leiden: Brill, 2009). It is very possible that some of these words originate from an old women from Crete, who is mentioned in the final section of paragraph 4 of the Preface, see f. 5v in print A and the corresponding passage in print B. Simon says that she taught him how to recognize plants and that she explained to him the properties of plants according to Dioscorides. This oral commentary tradition could also be behind other passages that do not explicitly cite a written source.

Certainly, Simon's critical first-hand accounts and assessments could be of help in identifying the actual plant, rather than risking tracking down a phantom that has been distorted in the many translations. However, for obvious reasons, we cannot tell the motives for accessing the website. Only some statistical data on the audience of *Simon Online* can be collected. Over the past year and a half, the project has attracted 662,756 page views (excluding bots) from 55,335 unique visitors in seventy-nine countries. The majority of these users access the site via the start page, presumably because they had bookmarked it at some point. Most likely, these users are in one way or another affiliated with medieval studies or the history of medicine, or following the e-mail lists associated with the field. Another, larger group, accesses lexicon entries through search engine requests, mainly via Google or Yandex, its Russian counterpart. Typically, these users would search for a medicinal plant or a product thereof.

At this point our analysis must, however, come to an end, as we do not know the motives of the readers. It can be said, however, that the website serves as a dictionary to the Latin, Greek, and Arabic medical and pharmaceutical terminology of the Middle Ages. In fact, even though it dates to the late thirteenth century, it is still the most comprehensive resource available. Most likely many readers have an interest in the history of medicine, or in lexicography. On the other hand, many of the words in the *Clavis* are still in use today, particularly plant names. It could well be the case that these Internet searches are motivated by an interest in contemporary herbal treatment.

*

It was clear from the outset that a project such as *Simon Online* would also need some form of intellectual property protection for the editors working on the website. The MediaWiki software we use is particularly suitable to track who wrote which part of the content displayed on the website: all contributions appear in the name of the respective author, including smaller edits; for instance: additions to the index. These data are displayed on the page itself and also on the user profiles. Moreover, we create an independent record that these pages in fact exist: all edited entries are being archived regularly on www.webcitation.org, a free service provided by the University of Toronto, that is suitable for dynamically changing content. The content on *Simon Online* is published under a Creative Commons license that excludes commercial exploitation and requires source attribution.[13]

---

[13] http://creativecommons.org/licenses/by-nc-nd/3.0/

Since the authorship of the entries can be tracked, it is also possible for the content to be listed on a CV. However, from my conversations with authors, there appears to be little interest in using contributions to *Simon Online* for career related purposes; for instance, by quoting them as a public engagement activity in research assessment exercises or grant applications. Rather, the main incentive for the authors appears to be the intellectual challenge, and providing information to the general public in an easily accessible way.

*

Altogether, the website is an open access research and publishing platform where progress can be viewed in real time. Currently, all of our authors have at least some background in Classics (although two now work as physicians), but we would also be interested in contributions from an entirely medical or pharmaceutical side, which could be done in collaboration with a philologist.

We now have reached a sufficient amount of edited entries, and have set up two gateways to the edition: one for Latin speakers, which brings up all entries including raw, unedited material; and one for those who prefer to read the text in English translation with a commentary. Users mainly navigate the website by clicking on menus and links, but it is also possible to type keywords such as 'bibliography', 'dictionaries', or 'index' in the search box in the right hand corner, followed by the enter key. This fast and easy method can also be used to browse for entries. For instance, typing the letter 'B' in the search box followed by the enter key brings up all available entries starting with this letter.

Many features of *Simon Online* can be used creatively; for instance, the index rerum is, in effect, also a reverse dictionary for English to Medieval Latin, Greek, or Arabic.

*

Looking back over the one and half years since its launch, *Simon Online* has certainly demonstrated that there is indeed a large readership for topics such as Medieval medicine, and that it is possible to introduce new ways of conducting research, namely in collaboration organized into a flowing system.

 The decision to open *Simon Online* to the public has been made because the topic was not compatible with the conventional way of editing. The fact that the content would also appear Open Access was an additional bonus. When looking at the academic publishing landscape as it presents today, it is felt that other, more conventional forms of research output could also benefit from an open access format, and here in particular books and collected essay volumes. Publishing the equivalent of an academic book series online is trivial from a technical point of view, and it would involve negligible costs. The most important parts of the work (research, writing, formatting, quality control, and, in many cases, editing) are already being carried out by academics. It would only be a very small step to set up branding, advertising, the IT framework, and a preservation plan. Powerful tools, such as search engines, index content free of charge and very quickly. A move towards online publication would not only make our work available straight away, it would also reach all those who are unable to access the (very few) well-funded research libraries available.

Bibliography

Dahhaoui, Yann, *L'atelier de Simon de Genes. Vers une edition de la Clavis Sanationis.* (MA thesis, Lausanne, 2001).

Riddle, John M. "Oral Contraceptives and Early-Term Abortifacients during Classical Antiquity and the Middle Ages", *Past and Present* 132 (1991, August), 3-32.

von Staden, Heinrich, *Herophilus. The Art of Medicine in Early Alexandria.* Cambridge: Cambridge University Press, 1989.

Zipser, Barbara, *John the Physician's Therapeutics: A Medical Handbook in Vernacular Greek.* Leiden: Brill, 2009.

General Index

Simon of Genoa's **Medical Lexicon**

1

1001 Nights 60

A

Abraham of Tortosa 11-12, 34, 62
Abulcasis 34, 36, 57
Acantis egyptia 104, 105, 110, 122, 124
Accursino of Pistoia 22
Acros 112, 115, 116
Adam of Kircudbright 21
Aëtius of Amida 112
Al-Andalus 94
Albenmesue 57
Albertus Magnus 20
Al-Bitriq 137-139, 142
Alchemy 22, 25-26
Alcohol 24
Alderotti, Taddeo 19, 26
Aleppo 13, 150
Alexander II 17
Alexander of Tralles 11, 35, 41, 99-128
Al-Jazzar 129
Al-Majūsī 57-58, 67, 70
Almansor 58
Alphita 101-102, 110-112
Al-Razi See Rhazes
Alum 55
Amitrocera 112-114, 116
Ambergris 55
Amnesia 24
Amphibians 37

Anagni 18
Anatomy 21-22
Animal origin 37
Anise 59, 150
Ant 150
Antelope 150
Antichrist 150
Antidotarium Nicolai 32, 45-46
Antioch 77
Anti-Popes 26
Anus 60
Aphrodisiac 150
Apothecary 32, 44
Apotropaic bells 26
Apple 150
Aquamarine 150
Aristotle 23
Arnald of Villanova 14-16, 18, 20- 22, 24
Ar-Rāzī See Rhazes
Arsenic 150
Artemisia 88, 137, 150
Arthomeli 124
Ashes 52
Astrologer 19, 34
Astrology 22, 26
Astronomy 21
Autopsy 26
Averroes 35, 58
Avicenna 23, 33, 36, 58-61, 93, 129, 142, 144
Avignon 24-25

Index of Manuscripts

Simon of Genoa's **Medical Lexicon**

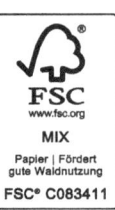

Zeitfracht Medien GmbH
Ferdinand-Jühlke-Straße 7
99095 Erfurt, Deutschland
produktsicherheit@kolibri360.de